The Fertility Doctor's Guide to
OVERCOMING INFERTILITY

The Fertility Doctor's Guide to

OVERCOMING INFERTILITY

Discovering Your Reproductive Potential
and Maximizing Your Odds of Having a Baby

Mark P. Trolice, M.D.

Director, Fertility CARE: The IVF Center

HARVARD
COMMON
PRESS

First Published in 2020 by The Harvard Common Press, an imprint of The Quarto Group, 100 Cummings Center, Suite 265-D, Beverly, MA 01915, USA.
T (978) 282-9590 F (978) 283-2742 QuartoKnows.com

The Harvard Common Press titles are also available at discount for retail, wholesale, promotional, and bulk purchase. For details, contact the Special Sales Manager by email at specialsales@quarto.com or by mail at The Quarto Group, Attn: Special Sales Manager, 100 Cummings Center, Suite 265-D, Beverly, MA 01915, USA.

23 22 21 20 24   1 2 3 4 5

ISBN: 978-1-55832-958-4

Digital edition published in 2020
eISBN: 978-1-55832-936-2

Library of Congress Cataloging-in-Publication Data is available.

Design: Elizabeth Van Itallie
Illustration: Shutterstock.com

Printed in China

The information in this book is for educational purposes only. It is not intended to replace the advice of a physician or medical practitioner. Please see your health-care provider before beginning any new health program.

Dedicated to my wife, Andrea,
the woman who taught me the true meaning of love and family.

Contents

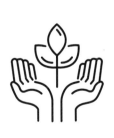

Foreword

BY BRENDA STRONG

National Spokesperson and Honorary Board Chair of
Path2Parenthood and Emmy-nominated actress

For eight wonderful years, I narrated the hit ABC show *Desperate Housewives* as the disembodied voice of Mary Alice, the character who took her life in the first episode but continued to illuminate the audience via her series-long voiceovers and flashbacks about her life and the lives of her friends on Wisteria Lane. The backstory for my character—as written by Marc Cherry, the executive producer and creator of *Desperate Housewives*—explained how Mary Alice became so desperate from infertility that she bought a child from a heroin-addicted woman in a treatment center where she worked.

Years later, once that woman had cleaned up her act, she came back to get her child. Out of protection and panic, Mary Alice accidentally killed that woman and, driven by shame and fear, she covered up the murder. Then, as the truth was about to be blackmailed out of her, she took her own life, which is how the series got off to a "bang" and thereby established the theme, which is that everyone has "dirty little secrets." Ironically, what Marc Cherry didn't know was that much like my character, I was secretly suffering from secondary infertility. Fortunately, my desperation led me to a much better place.

I had been teaching yoga for years alongside my acting career and had developed a proprietary approach to combat the stress of infertility using yoga. My specific approach also helps the reproductive area by improving circulation, reducing tension in the muscles and tissues in and around the pelvis, and aiding in hormonal balance.

Strong Yoga4Fertility was born out of my own pain and purpose to help empower women like me find a way to face the uncertainties of the fertility journey. I have helped thousands of women reduce their stress while trying to conceive, resulting in countless pregnancies worldwide: some on natural cycles and some with the help of their reproductive specialists. In all it has been my honor and privilege to play a small part in the fulfillment of helping so many couples realize their dreams of parenthood.

My passion for helping make even more of a difference then led me to Dr. Mark Trolice. I have seen firsthand that Dr. Trolice is an amazingly empathetic and empowering physician in the field of fertility. When I was first introduced to Dr. Trolice, he invited me to give a keynote speech at his Fertile Dreams Conference where, each year, Dr. Trolice gifted a couple with the funds to pursue free in vitro fertilization treatments.

It's not until something like an infertility diagnosis occurs that many of us are informed about the reproductive process and our chances to conceive—which points out how little, we as human beings, truly understand our bodies and how they function.

The sad truth is, we spend most of our lives as young adults trying *not* to get pregnant, so by the time we are ready, we are shocked to find out our bodies might have missed our prime fertility years. Pursuing careers, finding the right partner, and feeling emotionally prepared, oftentimes leaves us with a diminished ovarian reserve, stress, and a less than favorable fertile environment.

Of course Hollywood has not helped by promoting stories of actresses in their early to late 40s getting pregnant; albeit, without the overt explanation that their babies were most likely born via costly IVF and a possible egg donor. Our reproductive window is smaller than we know, and I have heard countless women ask, "Why didn't anyone tell me?!"

We are trying. We are trying to educate and inform women and couples about the cost of infertility financially, emotionally, and physically in order to hopefully head off the challenges on the road ahead.

That's why I got involved with fertility awareness and education, and that's why Dr. Trolice has written this book, which, without overwhelming you, provides the necessary knowledge and insight for you to go to your doctor feeling informed and ready to ask the right questions about your fertility.

In my 18-plus years of working with couples facing infertility and while serving as the National Spokesperson for The American Fertility Association (now called Path2Parenthood), I have worked alongside many of the best reproductive endocrinologists in the country, and rarely have I found such a devoted physician as Dr. Mark Trolice.

Perhaps some of that devotion is because he has also been a fertility patient. (I know that much of my drive comes from my personal experiences with infertility.) Such life-altering experiences have provided Dr. Trolice with the unique knowledge of the pain and disappointment that are unique to fertility struggles. In this book, he combines his professional and personal experience to provide you with the necessary tools that will guide you along the path from infertility to parenthood.

BRENDA STRONG is the national spokesperson for Path2Parenthood (www.path2parenthood.org) and currently serves on their board. Brenda is a Yoga Alliance certified 500 hr E-RYT who created the Strong Yoga4Fertility program to help women worldwide. She has taught at the Mind Body Institute at UCLA and Two Hearts Yoga and has licensed her trademarked Strong Yoga4Fertility program under Strong Yoga4Women (yoga4women.com). Brenda has been featured in Alternative Medicine magazine, Shape magazine, For Pregnancy, Plum, Conceive, Yoga Journal, *and* Yoga Magazine.

She is a two-time Emmy-nominated and award-winning actress, holds a BM from Arizona State University (magna cum laude), is a certified prenatal teacher, and was Miss Arizona 1980 in the Miss America Pageant. She serves on the board of Events of the Heart, a nonprofit organization assisting in women's heart disease education. Brenda is also the honorary recipient of a doctorate of science from Yo San University, specializing in Traditional Chinese Medicine, for her pioneering work in yoga for fertility.

Preface

Physicians are healers and teachers. When I meet with you as my patient, my purpose is to relieve your suffering and level the playing field by talking the same language. How? Through education of reproductive biology in simple terms and by sharing with you my ten-year personal journey and discovery of infertility. You see, your story is my story.

I have lived your lives and am committed to empowering you with this book. For ten long years, my wife and I endured the pain of infertility while I was a fertility specialist. Quite the irony, to be sure! (In case you are wondering, I chose and fell in love with the field of infertility way before we were diagnosed with infertility.) Throughout this book, I will share my insights from our personal challenge, from actual patient interactions, and at the same time, provide you a comprehensive and credible resource for all your reproductive questions and goals.

One of my major points of the book is to help you be your own advocate and be proactive with your fertility care. Rule #1 to #10, if your fertility clinic's behavior worsens your stress, it's time to move on to another clinic. Your path will usually have bumps (mine sure did!) of various sizes: Being told your insurance will cover a treatment and now it will not; the clinic has not returned your phone call and you are supposed to start medication; running out of ovarian stimulating medication and it's the weekend; and so on and so on. These are the bumps that may be flattened by a heart-to-heart talk with your fertility clinic regarding your grievances or by finding a clinic more suitable to your needs.

Bumps can also present as emotions, in the form of one or more of the following—feeling isolated, overwhelmed, being broken and less of a woman or man, failure, frustration, anger, sorrow, disappointment, regret, and anxiety. These emotions are entirely understandable and expected, but must be temporary because your journey toward success can begin only with acceptance of your current problem rather than continuing to deny the reality. A counselor, typically one who specializes in reproductive issues, may be required to assist you and facilitate moving forward. The mind/body connection is an integral part of my approach to your care, and I will explore this further with you in this book.

This book is not afraid to tell the truth about the potential conflict of physicians' interests and the risk of exploitation involved in treating infertility patients. My intention is to expose medical offers for which you must be cautious. Your desperation may make you susceptible to a greater, but unnecessary, financial burden.

My goal is for you to use this book as a companion on every step of your journey—a companion that explains the most optimal time to conceive, advises the right time for an evaluation by a fertility specialist, recommends evidence-based diagnostic testing and treatment, and discusses alternative family building such as egg/sperm donation, surrogacy, and adoption. These steps and more are fully addressed in the chapters that follow.

I sincerely hope my personal experience as a fertility patient combined with my professional experience as a fertility specialist will provide you with guidance, support, and encouragement to help you on your road to parenthood.

CHAPTER 1

The Music of Medicine

Growing up, I adored my parents and had an innate desire to please them through my grades and my music. My dad was a professional musician and entertainer. He took great pride in teaching me how to perform onstage in front of a live audience. From my mother, I inherited genes from a long line of classical musicians and opera singers. In my family, love of performing meant no crowd was too small and no event was too trivial. Music and singing remain vital parts of my life.

And, just as music has always been there, so too has medicine. At age eleven, one summer afternoon, I was running with my cousins through my aunt's house when I accidentally put my hand through a glass door. At the emergency room later that day, my escalating fear of receiving stitches on my hand turned to a calm curiosity; I just had to watch the doctor work on my hand. Everyone was amazed by my behavior, including me. On that day, my passion for medicine was born, and it has never waned.

No doctors had ever emerged from my family, so my role models were the dedicated physicians who treated my family. The cardiologist, who transformed my father—a stubborn, overweight Italian smoker—into a compliant patient. The general practitioner, who, as my mother would say with conviction, ". . . is the best because he answers all questions with patience and understanding." These were some of my earliest inspirations and to whom I remain indebted.

That "A-ha" Moment

Fast forward to my senior year at Columbia University on a chilly spring morning when my two worlds collided. During one of my medical school interviews in New York City, I was asked about my life's purpose. I confidently and sincerely conveyed my passion for helping others and declared the pursuit of medicine as a calling to my vocation. Likewise, that conversation turned to other interests of mine including, naturally, music. My eyes gave it away. Thirty years later, I vividly remember and regret my stumbling attempt to answer one simple question, "If you love music to this degree, why are you pursuing a medical career?" I was stumped!

Not only was I unable to convince the medical school interviewer that I loved medicine more than music, to this day I am unable to convince myself. Which brings us to my epiphany moment. Why does one have to choose? Following years of an internal tug of war, I have learned from personal experience—and from the multitude of research findings on the relationships between arts and medicine—that these two worlds not only harmoniously coexist, but that I am a better physician because of my musical side.

In other words, because I perform as a singer (under the stage name of Mark Romeo), my "day job" as a physician is noticeably improved by my musical experiences.

While I will admit that singing onstage in front of a jazz band is not for everyone, many other creative expressions have been proven to enhance doctors' relationships and effectiveness with their patients. For example, research shows that a physician with an inclination for poetry is more likely to be better at their job because, as doctors Jack Coulehan and Patrick Clary have written, "Reading and writing poetry can help physicians, especially those who care for dying patients, become more reflective, creative, and compassionate practitioners." In the movie *Dead Poets Society*, Professor John Keating, played brilliantly by the late Robin Williams, best defines the coexisting worlds of art and medicine: "We don't read and write poetry because it's cute. We read and write poetry because we are members of the human race. And the human race is filled with passion. And medicine, law, business, engineering, these are noble pursuits and necessary to sustain life. But poetry, beauty, romance, love, these are what we stay alive for. To quote from Whitman, 'O me! O life! Of the questions of these recurring, of the endless trains of the faithless, of cities filled with the foolish. What good amid these, O me, O life? Answer. That you are here—that life exists, and identity, that the powerful play goes on, and you may contribute a verse.' That the powerful play goes on and you may contribute a verse. What will your verse be?"

My verse came to me during my third year as a medical student. While being exposed to every disease and specialty in rapid succession, I experienced the fabled "a-ha" moment. It was during my obstetrics and gynecology (OB/GYN) course rotation, and at once, those five days of observing and interacting with fertility patients transformed me from outsider to insider.

Clinging to their dreams, couples expressed a myriad of emotions from happiness to sorrow mixed with anger and frustration in a seemingly perpetual cycle. The feelings of connection and compassion I felt that day were both compelling and comforting, and they continue undeterred through today.

Ironically, my attachment and passion for this field were the prelude to a more profound experience, in which I would soon learn that while procreation is a simple reflex for some, it is a complex and insurmountable goal for others.

The Wrong Side of the Playground Fence

Upon graduating medical school, my soulmate and I were married. We were young and free of any fertility risk factors, so why wouldn't it be easy for us? In the middle of an arduous four-year OB/GYN residency, our family building plans were placed on hold. Due to long hours at the hospital, our dedication to ovulation-timed intercourse was replaced on our "spare time priority list" by sleep, eat, sleep, and more sleep. In year three, as residency training demands eased, we committed to building our family, and so my wife discontinued contraception as we segued from having relations exclusively for intimacy, to the purpose of having a child. After one year of conception attempts, we painfully accepted the reality of infertility—we became part of the roughly 12 percent of couples in the United States experiencing infertility.

Without justification, I was pessimistic about our fertility future just one month into our journey. This negativity didn't help our mood—something that many patients have described as a sixth sense of their own infertility. We persevered and months turned into two years almost overnight. Despite using ovulation predictor kits and making awkward excuses to my colleagues for urgent "home visits," we were unable to conceive naturally. Suddenly, we were faced with the same crisis as every patient I would eventually encounter in my fertility clinic. Unfortunately, the experience included the unrelenting questions from family, friends, and each other. Isolating, biologically assaulting, and sexually paralyzing, fertility issues became the unspoken voice of our lives.

Though I resisted every consideration of fertility treatment, my wife won every discussion. I accepted this continuous defeat by rationalizing the parental invest- ment—maternal is emphatically different from paternal. Time began to fly and stand still simultaneously. Every intrauterine insemination cycle (IUI) accelerated the high of our expectations but two weeks later, a negative pregnancy test brought despair. The peaks and valleys began to run more parallel than divergent. We told no one, at least not for many years. Work schedules became the excuse not to attend family gatherings or children's birthdays to avoid the painful reminder of our void. Several unsuccessful years of treatment led to in vitro fertilization, despite our denial and disbelief. Would we ever enjoy the laughter of our own children or be relegated to the wrong side of the playground fence? Our faces became pressed up against the windows of families and the glass seemed impenetrable.

Our silver lining was my wife's unabated optimism and tenacity to have a family despite the multiple failed attempts over ten years. Through her eyes, I found the hope and promise of a family. For what is a family if not simply people who grow in the same home and love each other? Our choice became, "Would we allow the years of struggle to define us or ensure our destiny through all means available?" Ultimately my epiphany was the realization that no one's life develops as planned. My lifelong axiom of faith became, "It's not how you start but how you finish."

Originally not a proponent of adoption, I found myself overjoyed when our daugh- ter's birth mother matched with us. When I held our little angel for the first time, I knew she was born in our hearts and meant to be ours. She was chosen. The same miracle occurred the next time when we adopted our son. Despite the onerous ten years, I would immediately repeat the entire pursuit for the reward of my five precious children—all adopted, all chosen, all born in our hearts.

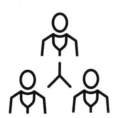

Contributing My Own Verse

And so we jumped over the fence, onto the playground and became a family. What I have learned from our journey is the plans and ideas we had when we were younger will change. Nevertheless, our true character and integrity emerge when we face adversity and overcome our challenge to find fulfillment, not necessarily in the manner we originally intended.

Ping Fu, in her 2013 book, *Bend, Not Break: A Life in Two Worlds*, explained it best: "Bamboo is flexible, bending with the wind but never breaking, capable of adapting to any circumstance. It suggests resilience, meaning that we have the ability to bounce back even from the most difficult times. Your ability to thrive depends, in the end, on your attitude to your life circumstances. Take everything in stride with grace, putting forth energy when it is needed, yet always staying calm inwardly."

Every day, I venture out into both of my worlds, not in conflict but cooperative. Physician/musician, surgeon/performer . . . yet, always a healer/teacher, applying all my talent to ease the burden of my patients and my audience, while soothing their minds and contributing my own verse.

Every one of you has your own story to tell; each is personal and unique. Mine involved the contradiction of treating infertility and, simultaneously, suffering infertility, 24/7. Who do we tell? Well, the only one who "gets" our story is someone else who has walked our walk. I vowed to never forget how it felt to be on the outside of the playground watching parents play with their children. That memory is part of what drives me ceaselessly to empower you with knowledge and offer guidance—so that one day, hopefully, you may share your story with a happy ending.

CHAPTER 2

First, Protect Your Fertility

How big of a problem is infertility? In addition to the 1 in 8 couples that have trouble getting pregnant or sustaining a pregnancy in the United States, about 50 million couples worldwide who are in the reproductive age group of 15 to 44 meet the definition of infertility. This represents an astounding 10 percent of women globally. Obviously a major health issue, infertility ranks high in importance for women and couples, which is precisely why I created the following series of priorities known as my **SWAT** analysis for protecting your fertility in much the same way a SWOT (Strengths, Weaknesses, Opportunities, and Threats) analysis is used to protect a business.

SWAT stands for fertility's four vital risk areas: Sexually transmitted infections/ **S**tress, **W**eight, **A**ge, **T**obacco. Each area has a profound negative impact on both female and male infertility.

Sexually Transmitted Infections (STIs)

STIs usually result from gonorrhea or chlamydia and are, what I like to call, the "silent-killers" of fertility. Most infections from these bacteria are without symptoms but can wreak havoc on your fallopian tubes and surrounding pelvic organs. STI symptoms are typically mild and include vaginal discharge with odor and burning on urination. Left untreated, STIs can result in abdominal and pelvic pain and fever as well as the potential for hospitalization due to PID (pelvic inflammatory disease). With PID, the endometrium (lining of the uterus) becomes infected, called endometritis, as do the fallopian tubes, called salpingitis, resulting in a hydrosalpinx (blocked swollen end of the fallopian tube filled with fluid; for more information, see chapter 10). Further risk is the surrounding organs becoming covered in scar tissue and tubal factor infertility (TFI). Each case of PID dramatically worsens the chance for TFI.

By not practicing safer sex, specifically, barrier contraception, you may be placing yourself at risk for TFI and/or an ectopic pregnancy (a pregnancy outside the uterus and often in the fallopian tube). The latter complication occurs in 2 percent of all pregnancies but increases to 8 percent after a prior PID infection. The incidence of TFI increases seven-fold, 16-fold, and 28-fold, following one, two, and three infections to the fallopian tubes, respectively. Aggressive screening and prompt treatment may reduce the damage to reproductive potential.

Stress

A topic that deserves its own chapter, and maybe its own book, stress and fertility will forever be etched in the minds of all those amateur reproductive specialists generously offering, unsolicited, their diagnosis and treatment of infertility to you. How many times have you shared your problem of infertility and been advised to, "Just relax so it will happen?" Not only have laypeople offered this advice but, unfortunately, you all have also been subjected to this baseless suggestion by physicians, just as generations of fertility patients before you were.

Having said that, stress does play a role in infertility. A recent study looked at a stress hormone called salivary alpha-amylase (SAA) in women trying to conceive (TTC) for one year. The findings were: (1) 29 percent of women who had the higher levels of SAA took a longer time to conceive; and (2) women with the highest SAA levels had a 12 percent less likely chance to conceive each month.

My criticisms of such results include (1) SAA is not always involved in stress, (2) using saliva is not always an accurate method of testing, and (3) cortisol, the major stress hormone, levels were unaffected.

Nonetheless, it is definitive that infertility can cause stress and there is some research that stress, specifically depression, may increase the risk of infertility. Please recognize that infertility is a challenge and you may find comfort in speaking with a counselor who has expertise in this area.

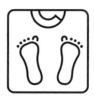

Weight

Twelve percent of all infertility cases can be attributed to women being either overweight or even underweight. For men, obesity can reduce fertility, too.

In the United States, nearly 40 percent of the population are obese. This is a major health problem with risks of cardiovascular disease, diabetes, as well as infertility. A common hormonal abnormality often associated with an elevated body mass index (BMI—a measure of body fat based on height and weight) is Polycystic Ovary Syndrome (PCOS), which can lead to an ovulation disorder (more on this in chapter 13). In men, obesity results in a hormonal disturbance causing decreased testosterone and sperm counts by increased estrogen production in fat cells. The higher levels of estrogen feedback on the brain's pituitary gland and reduces the release of follicle stimulating hormone (FSH), a hormone needed for sperm production.

You can also be too thin. An extremely low BMI can affect ovulation and is often seen with the very common (but not well-known) Female Athlete Triad of amenorrhea, bone loss, and eating disorder. (See chapter 7: Optimizing Women's Prenatal Health.) An eating disorder is estimated in 15 to 62 percent of female college athletes.

According to the American Society for Reproductive Medicine (ASRM), an optimal BMI is key to your healthy reproduction: A BMI above 175 percent of ideal body weight results in menstrual irregularity. Fortunately, over 70 percent of obese infertile women with ovulation dysfunction will conceive spontaneously with an average weight loss of 10 kg (22 pounds).

Even if you conceive with an elevated BMI, you remain at risk for higher pregnancy complications for you and baby—including miscarriage, gestational diabetes and hypertension, preeclampsia, preterm delivery, stillbirth, cesarean delivery, shoulder dystocia complicating a vaginal delivery, fetal distress, early baby's death, and small-for-gestational-age (as well as large-for-gestational-age) infants.

Age

The average age of first-time mothers continues to advance globally. In the United States, this age began rapidly advancing in the 1970s. Women delay childbearing usually due to the lack of a partner but also for career reasons. To be sure, the problem of ovarian aging, namely, diminished ovarian reserve (DOR), is increasing. The main impact on pregnancy rate is oocyte (egg) quality and quantity. As a result, fertilization is negatively affected, implantation is reduced, and miscarriage is increased.

So you can understand DOR, let's look at its two components—the quality of eggs and quantity of eggs. The term *quality* as it relates to the egg is a nebulous description because there are no clear-cut criteria. While embryologists love to view an embryo that appears perfect in shape (morphology), this evaluation alone has a limited correlation with pregnancy. Rather, chromosomal analysis of the embryo preimplantation is considered the best measure of quality and is the best prediction of embryo implantation. Quality of eggs is based on your birthday—the more birthdays, the poorer the quality. Actually, egg quality begins to decline after you pass age 30. Quantity, on the other hand, is determined indirectly by the result of a hormone blood test and a pelvic ultrasound.

Ovarian aging is currently best measured by considering three things: your chronologic age; your antral follicle count (AFC), small ovarian cysts with immature eggs that can be measured with a pelvic ultrasound; and your levels of Anti-Müllerian hormone (AMH), which can be assessed with a blood test. Natural fertility begins to decline on average above age of 30 for a woman. An AFC less than eleven reflects DOR, and less than six is severe DOR. Low AMH levels, defined as below 1 nanogram per milliliter of blood, have been shown to reduce the number of eggs retrieved with IVF and may predict pregnancy outcome. AMH levels below 0.4 ng/mL are severe.

The use of a screening test for DOR in a random population at low risk for infertility will result in a larger number of false-positive results (i.e., saying a woman has DOR when in fact she has a normal ovarian reserve).

Very low AMH levels (less than or equal to 0.4) affect the outcome of IVF cycles as a woman ages. I can explain, in 2016 the *Journal Fertility & Sterility* reported data using the Society for Assisted Reproductive Technology (SART) statistics. The women had a mean age of 39.4 years and were treated with IVF. Due to a poor ovarian response to stimulating medication, 54 percent of women were cancelled prior to egg retrieval. In those who underwent an egg-retrieval attempt, no eggs were obtained in

5.4 percent of patients and no embryo transfer occurred in 25.1 percent of cycles. The live birth rate per embryo transfer was 20.5 percent (9.5 percent per cycle start and 16.3 percent per retrieval) occurring in women with a mean age of 36.8 years.

In a nutshell, random screening of AMH levels in women not diagnosed with infertility and less than 35 years of age may result in unnecessary alarm. While it is possible the results of AMH screening may encourage you to electively freeze your eggs, I recommend extensive counseling on the realistic implications of the number of eggs you will obtain if you have a low AMH level. There is no current evidence that AMH levels should be used to exclude patients from undergoing IVF.

According to the ASRM, the review of medical studies on ovarian reserve tests have limited value due to a small number of patients, different types of study design and analysis, and a lack of valid tools to measure outcomes.

Bottom Line: Your best chance for a pregnancy is attempting to conceive before your 30th birthday.

For so many years, all fertility physicians believed men can father a child indefinitely. More recently, however, males over the age of 40 have been shown to have an increased risk of infertility and miscarriage, as well as offspring with a higher rate of birth defect, schizophrenia, and autism. While this data is preliminary, certainly further studies are vital due to the current trend of delaying parenting in both men and women.

Given all this, I am broaching the topic more frequently with my male patients and encouraging, but not requiring, them to freeze their sperm if they are childless or infertile and approaching 40.

Tobacco

Approximately one-third of all men and women in the United States smoke cigarettes, which has made tobacco responsible for 13 percent of infertility cases. This behavior (even half a pack per day) results in a 40 to 60 percent increase in infertility. Cigarette smoking, including second-hand smoke, accelerates the loss of eggs and results in higher rates of miscarriages, ectopic pregnancies, an earlier onset of menopause, and possible genetic damage to eggs and sperm. If that's not bad enough, when compared to nonsmokers, female smokers have a reduced ovarian reserve; a less positive ovarian response to fertility medication; and a lower number of eggs retrieved and fertilized in IVF. To top it off, the pregnancy rate in IVF treatment cycles is decreased in smokers by 34 percent!

In male smokers, sperm counts are reduced an average of 22 percent and will worsen with increased cigarette smoking. Even when sperm counts remain in the normal range, smoking reduces sperm fertilization potential.

The good news is that within a year of stopping smoking, you may be able to return to normal fertility.

In other words: If you do not smoke, please don't begin. If you or your partner smoke, the smoking needs to stop in order to improve your fertility. Just think—what would you rather be holding, a cigarette or a baby?

Five Misconceptions to Avoid

REFRAIN FROM INTERCOURSE UNTIL OVULATION

In all my years of being a fertility specialist, I never corrected an infertility couple for having too much intercourse! In other words, the more relations, the more optimal timing for conception. And while you may be thinking "duh," you will be surprised (or maybe not) at the amount of misinformation given to couples TTC naturally.

Not a day goes by in my office where I am reminded how optimal timing of reproduction is so confusing for my patients. Many times after I point out the ideal days for intercourse, the husband and wife turn to each other and say, "we've been doing it wrong."

First things first. Get a cheap, over-the-counter, urine ovulation predictor kit (OPK). Meaning? No thousand-dollar electronically sensitive OPK; no basal body temperature (BBT) charting; no mobile apps, No Apps, NO APPS! Using an inexpensive OPK, you will learn the approximate onset of your brain's luteinizing hormone (LH) surge resulting in ovulation within 24 to 36 hours. Your prime time for "hooking-up" is the day before, day of, and day after the LH surge. If your cycles are monthly, this optimal window will become clearer to you.

Second, you should not abstain from intercourse to increase sperm counts at ovulation because abstinence will only decrease the quality of the first ejaculate. Perform relations daily to no further apart than every other day over the three days prior to ovulation to improve the chance of conception.

INFERTILITY IS RARE

In fact, infertility is not at all rare. In the United States alone, here are some telling statistics:

- Women aged 15 to 44 with infertility: 6.1 million or 10 percent
- Married women aged 15 to 44 that are infertile: 6.7 percent
- Women ages 15 to 44 who have ever used infertility services: 7.3 million or 12 percent

FORTY AND FERTILE

While conception can certainly be achieved if either of you are above the age of 39, fertility declines with age due to the loss of your egg/sperm number and quality. As a result, time to conceive is longer and the miscarriage rate is higher as you age. If you are a man at this age, reproduction not only declines but there is an increased risk of miscarriage, preterm birth, birth defects, autism, and schizophrenia in offspring.

THE "BLAME GAME"

Having difficulty conceiving, one or both of you are certainly susceptible to stress to varying degrees and you usually handle it differently. A serious concern to your relationship stability is if you presume the problem is with your partner.

Despite common opinion, in a male-female couple the causes of infertility are divided equally among both of you (40 percent each, with the other 20 percent being unexplained). The most common obstacles found in women who have difficulty conceiving are tubal blockage and ovulation disorders. For men, your fertility is usually first evaluated with a routine sperm analysis unless there are predisposing factors such as prior treatment of cancer. A counselor experienced in reproductive health can be a valuable resource to you both while you are TTC.

This topic brings up a difficult consultation I experienced with a devastated couple who came to me as patients. During their first visit, the wife began crying and accusing the husband of causing their infertility due to his acquiring an STI during his prior marriage. While the infection was HPV (human papilloma virus) and not a known cause of infertility, this did not comfort the wife or reduce her anger. It was an uncomfortable consultation where I encouraged them both to explore their feelings and renew their reasons to build their family as well as to have a session with the reproductive psychologist who works at our clinic. We met for several subsequent consultations. They ultimately reconciled their animosity, realized the anger was over infertility, and agreed on dismissing the finger-pointing. Thankfully they conceived their daughter on the first cycle of IVF and conceived their second child on their next IVF cycle. When they now pass our office, their joy and love are immeasurable.

GOING TO A FERTILITY SPECIALIST IS A LAST RESORT

Plain and simple: The sooner you see a reproductive endocrinology and infertility (REI) specialist, the shorter the time to pregnancy. If you are less than 35 years of age, an evaluation is recommended following one year of TTC when there are no other factors such as abnormal menstrual cycles or prior cancer therapy in the male or female. In you are over 35 years of age, an evaluation is recommended following six months of TTC or after three months of conception attempts if you are above age 39. The change in recommended time for an evaluation is simply due to advancing ovarian age decreasing fertility rates.

Today IVF is the most successful treatment option available to those of you experiencing infertility. Not only are pregnancy rates significantly higher than fertility medication combined with intrauterine insemination (IUI) (for more information on IUI, see chapter 17: Reproductive Procedures), but clinics can now offer embryo testing for genetic disorders, chromosomal abnormalities such as Down syndrome, and family balancing with gender determination—all performed while the embryo is in the laboratory (i.e., preimplantation). Additionally, when there are excess embryos, you have the option of freezing them for future pregnancy attempts and for fertility preservation to maintain the biologic age of your eggs at the time of freezing.

In Conclusion

While most people are born fertile, your lifestyle and choices can impact your ultimate ability to conceive. Employing my SWAT analysis and correcting the above myths, you will have the best chance for conception. Knowledge is not only power, it's a necessity!

CHAPTER 3

Optimizing Women's Prenatal Health

In 2011, an enlightening report in the *New England Journal of Medicine* revealed that nearly half of all pregnancies in the United States were unintended. Among these unintended pregnancies, 42 percent ended in abortion. Why would I begin a chapter in an infertility book about unintended pregnancies and abortion? Well, before you begin to think I have gone off track, let me regain your trust. As a lifelong advocate of women's health, I believe an unplanned pregnancy is analogous to an unprepared pregnancy. Unless a woman or couple address the important issues that I discuss below, the pregnancy and baby are at risk of significant negative outcomes.

The desire to have a child is one of the most powerful and consuming pursuits a woman experiences in her life. Yet I see a high percentage of patients who are not medically prepared for their pregnancy. This is not to isolate the fault of the woman. Their primary physician, OB/GYN, and even fertility specialist may prescribe fertility medication without fully stressing the need to optimize a woman's health prior to conception—without encouraging her to be prepared to be pregnant, in other words.

The more optimal your health is prior to pregnancy, the more likely you will experience a healthy pregnancy and baby. During the first 8 weeks of pregnancy, your baby is growing rapidly and developing its vital organs. Any compromise to your health and nutrition during this critical stage can risk your baby's growth and development.

So what exactly should a woman start doing early to ensure a healthy pregnancy?

— Get proper nutrition.
— Improve her BMI by exercising more, for example.
— Make sure she has the proper immunizations (typically rubella/MMR, tetanus, flu, varicella/chicken pox).
— Discontinue substance abuse (tobacco, alcohol, drugs).
— Stabilize any medical condition and make sure any current prescription and OTC medications will be safe during pregnancy; a simple Google search of the drug's name plus the word pregnancy will alert you to a drug's safety during pregnancy (see below).

CATEGORY	RISK
Category A	These are the safest drugs to take during pregnancy— No known adverse reactions.
Category B	No risks have been found in humans.
Category C	Not enough research has been done to determine if these drugs are safe.
Category D	Adverse reactions have been found in humans.
Category X	Should never be used by a pregnant woman

— Determine if you and/or your partner have a family history of an inheritable (genetic) disease (more on this in chapter 19: Embryo Testing and Genetics).
— Assess toxic environmental exposure at home and/or workplace (for example: lead or mercury, chemicals such as pesticides or solvents, or radiation).

Health Checks to Have Before Becoming a Parent

An expecting mom wants the best for the delicate new life developing in her womb. However, many couples are not aware that the health of both parents plays a key role both before conception and throughout pregnancy. The health of the mother-to-be especially is intricately linked to the health of the fetus throughout the pregnancy.

According to the ACOG, all women planning to have a child should undergo a preconception checkup. This enables your OB/GYN to determine whether there are issues that could negatively impact you or your baby's health and correct these issues to optimize the outcome.

The most critical health factors for prospective parents are

— Diet and lifestyle
— Current medications
— Updating vaccinations
— Medical and family history

How Can You Ensure Your Diet Is Healthy?

While no food affects your fertility, positively or negatively, extremes of body weight for the woman and obesity for the man undoubtedly impair your reproductive capability. Approximately 12 percent of all infertility cases can be attributed to women being either overweight or underweight.

To illustrate, let's consider the Female Athlete Triad, a potentially life-threatening disorder represented by three components: a low calorie intake with reduced energy availability; menstrual irregularity; and decreased bone mineral density. Not all cases of energy deficit result from eating disorders (i.e., anorexia and bulimia). Menstrual irregularity is due to a disruption of signals from the brain to the ovaries. The most common menstrual disorder seen in this triad is amenorrhea (lack of periods). Lastly, bone loss occurs because the lack of normal signals reduces the amount of estrogen production by the ovaries that is vital to maintain bone density. In a study of high school female athletes, 18.2 percent, 23.5 percent, and 21.8 percent met the criteria for disordered eating, menstrual irregularity, and low bone mass, respectively. Ten girls (5.9 percent) met criteria for 2 components of the triad, and 2 girls (1.2 percent) met criteria for all 3 components.

In men, obesity results in a hormonal disturbance causing a reduction in testosterone and sperm counts.

The Journal of the American Medical Association (called *JAMA* for short) recently indicated that nearly 40 percent of American adults were obese in 2015 and 2016, a sharp increase from a decade earlier. The Mediterranean Diet stresses plant-based foods and has been shown to increase success with IVF. In 2018 it was selected as the healthiest overall diet by *US News & World Report*.

KEY COMPONENTS OF THE MEDITERRANEAN DIET

- Plant-based foods, such as fruits and vegetables, whole grains, legumes, and nuts
- Healthy fats such as olive oil and canola oil (not butter!)
- Using herbs and spices for food flavoring (not salt!)
- Limiting red meat and replacing with chicken, duck, and turkey
- Increasing fish, such as trout, herring, sardines, and salmon are great sources of omega-3 fatty acids (avoid high mercury fish such as mackerel and tuna during pregnancy)
- Moderate amounts of red wine (avoid absolutely all alcohol while pregnant)

I am very excited about promoting this diet for prepregnancy health. While there is no diet definitively shown to increase your chance of having a baby naturally, recent evidence suggests the Mediterranean Diet may improve outcome with fertility treatment, specifically following IVF treatment, even in nonobese women. Men may also benefit from this diet, whether or not they're obese, to improve sperm health, sperm concentration, total sperm count, and sperm motility.

What Vitamins and Minerals Should You Take Prior to Conception?

Vitamins and minerals play important roles in all body functions. A daily prenatal vitamin (PNV) and a well-rounded diet provide all the vitamins and minerals needed during pregnancy. A vital component in PNV is folic acid, which is a B vitamin. Before and during pregnancy, a woman requires a minimum of 400 micrograms (0.4 milligrams or mg) of folic acid daily to help prevent major congenital disabilities of the fetal brain and spine called neural tube defects. Most PNVs have up to 1 mg of folic acid, an amount which has also been shown to potentially improve fertility. Folic acid should be started at least three months before TTC. The American College of Obstetricians and Gynecologists (ACOG) recommends pregnant and lactating women have an average daily intake of at least 200 mg docosahexaenoic acid (DHA) a day in addition to their prenatal vitamins.

In addition to folic acid, during pregnancy, a woman needs about double the amount of iron than nonpregnant women. This helps a mother-to-be make more blood to carry oxygen to the baby. Most PNVs provide the daily amount of iron needed (27 mg). Iron-rich foods include

— Lean red meat
— Poultry
— Fish
— Dried beans and peas
— Iron-fortified cereals
— Prune juice

Calcium is also needed during pregnancy to build the baby's bones and teeth. All women, including pregnant women, aged 19 years and older, should receive 1,000 mg of calcium daily. Calcium food sources include milk and other dairy products, such as cheese and yogurt. For women who cannot tolerate milk, other sources include

— Broccoli
— Dark, leafy greens
— Sardines
— Calcium supplements

Vitamin D works with calcium to help the baby's bones and teeth develop. It also is essential for healthy skin and eyesight. All women, including those who are pregnant, need 600 international units of vitamin D per day. Good sources of vitamin D include

— Milk fortified with vitamin D
— Fatty fish such as salmon
— Sunlight exposure also converts a chemical in the skin to vitamin D

SUMMARY OF NUTRITIONAL RECOMMENDATIONS IN PREGNANCY
- Appropriate weight gain
- Consumption of a variety of primarily whole, unprocessed foods in amounts to ensure appropriate, but not excessive, weight gain
- Indicated vitamin and mineral supplementation
- Avoidance of alcohol, tobacco, and other harmful substances
- Safe food handling

Summary

— Make your grandmother proud and remember your fruits and vegetables.
— Switch to skim milk or 1% milk.
— Eat whole grains.
— Vary your protein sources. Eat fish 2 to 3 times a week and choose lean meats and poultry. Vegetarians can get protein from plant-based foods such as nuts, seeds, and soy products.
— Limit foods with "empty" calories. These are foods that have a lot of calories but little nutritional value, such as candy, chips, and sugary drinks.
— Take a vitamin supplement that contains 600 micrograms of folic acid and 27 mg of iron.

(American College of Obstetrics and Gynecology)

Can Your Lifestyle Affect Your Pregnancy?

Smoking, drinking alcohol, and using drugs can reduce your fertility and, if taken during pregnancy, can have harmful effects on a fetus. While the full extent of damage has not been determined, alcohol use during pregnancy can result in mental retardation of the baby (Fetal Alcohol Syndrome).

TOBACCO

Approximately one-third of all men and women in the United States smoke cigarettes. Smoking is responsible for 13 percent of cases of female infertility. Even when it does not lead to complete infertility, this behavior (even half of a pack per day) results in a 40 to 60 percent increase in infertility. Smoking (even second-hand smoke) accelerates the loss of eggs and can result in

— Higher rates of miscarriages
— Ectopic pregnancies
— Earlier onset of menopause
— Possible genetic damage to eggs and sperm

Males who smoke can see their sperm count diminish by an average of 22 percent as well as experience a decrease in sperm fertilization potential.

Do Existing Medical Conditions Affect Your Pregnancy?

Unstable medical conditions such as diabetes mellitus, high blood pressure, depression, and seizure disorders can cause problems during pregnancy. Therefore, attempts at conception should be deferred until your health is optimized. Uncontrolled medical conditions can result in significant harm to both mother and baby.

Medications used to treat disease may also harm the fetus. You can verify the harmful risk of any drug by checking its pregnancy category. Categories A and B are the safest to use while categories C and D progressively increase the risk to a baby. Category X is contraindicated during pregnancy. See Pregnancy Categories of Medications and Risks on page 28.

Can You Prevent Infections?

Vaccination (immunization) can prevent some infections, but some vaccines aren't safe to use during pregnancy. It's important to know which vaccines you may need and to get them before becoming pregnant.

The following vaccines are safe to be given during pregnancy:
— Tdap (tetanus, diphtheria, and pertussis)
— Influenza (inactivated)

The following vaccines should be avoided during pregnancy:
— MMR (measles, mumps, and rubella)
— Varicella (for chicken pox)
— Influenza (live attenuated)

The following antibody levels should be checked prior to pregnancy. If you are found to lack appropriate levels of antibodies to fight these infections, a simple vaccination can be obtained to protect you and your baby. Remember, an ounce of prevention is worth a pound of cure (quote attributed to Benjamin Franklin).
— Rubella
— Varicella

If a pregnant woman acquires rubella (the German measles), her baby is at risk of congenital rubella syndrome with the associated risks of
— Miscarriage
— Stillbirth
— Mental retardation
— Deafness

Chicken pox (varicella virus) during pregnancy risks life-threatening pneumonia for the mother. If varicella is acquired within the week of delivery, then the baby is at risk for a rare condition known as neonatal varicella syndrome that comes with potentially life-threatening complications.

Family Health History

Is it important for you and your partner to share your family health histories with your infertility healthcare professional? Absolutely. The best rule of thumb for any couple planning to start a family is know your genes!

Some health conditions occur more often in certain families or ethnic groups. These conditions are called genetic or inherited disorders. If a close relative has a specific disease, you or your baby could be at higher risk of having it. Over 100 genetic mutations can be tested in the couple TTC. If one member of the couple is a carrier (typically without symptoms) of a mutation, the baby's risk is limited to being a carrier. However, if both partners are carriers of the same genetic mutation, the baby has a 25 percent risk of inheriting the disease, which could possibly be life threatening depending on the illness.

Thanks to preimplantation genetic testing (PGT) and reproductive genetics (see chapter 19: Embryo Testing and Genetics), embryos can be screened for specific genetic diseases that either member of the couple is known to carry in order to avoid transference to the baby. PGT is "preimplantation" testing, that is, following an egg retrieval and fertilization of the eggs, an embryologist removes a small amount of tissue from each embryo for genetic analysis. The tested embryos are frozen and an embryo transfer is deferred to a subsequent cycle while waiting for the results. Alternatively, screening can be performed early on during an established pregnancy. These tests include analyzing mom's blood in the first trimester as well as using ultrasound to detect signs of abnormalities in the baby. If necessary, at the end of the first trimester, chorionic villus sampling (CVS), which requires the removal of a small of tissue from the baby's placenta, can be performed for a more detailed study of chromosomal (e.g., Down syndrome) and genetic disorders (e.g., cystic fibrosis, sickle cell) based on the baby's risk.

In Conclusion

One of, if not *the* most important decisions in your life is to have a baby. Adhering to this chapter's guidelines will allow you to optimize the outcome of you and your baby during pregnancy and beyond. Please discuss any questions you have with your OB/GYN prior to conception so you can be confident of the best preparation for a healthy pregnancy.

CHAPTER 4

Understanding Ovulation

M y first year of medical school was full of courses that taught me all that was normal in the human body—no cancer, no infection, just normal. Eager to get to some pathology to understand disease, I asked my professor when those courses would start. His answer has stayed with me these many years: "Mark, you can't understand abnormal until you master what's normal."

A New Day—The Menstrual Phase

All reproductive biology begins with mastering the menstrual cycle—that finely tuned orchestration of hormonal changes—the sole purpose of which is to establish a pregnancy. As years pass and I grow in my knowledge of the process of ovulation, I truly marvel at its synchrony, complexity, and elegance.

The first day of your ovulation cycle is referred to as Cycle Day One. It is the first day of full-flow menstrual bleeding and, simultaneously, ends one cycle while beginning the next—much in the same representation as our daily time of midnight.

The end of a cycle means no pregnancy has occurred, so the hormones that were preparing for an embryo to implant, mainly progesterone but also estradiol, decline. This withdrawal of hormones initiates the shedding of your uterine lining (the endometrium), hence your period flow.

At the start of your cycle, called the menstrual phase, your endometrium sheds and begins to heal due to estradiol production from the ovaries as a new cycle starts. You would continue to bleed if estradiol were not produced to stop your menstrual flow and rebuild your endometrium.

THE FIRST HALF—THE FOLLICULAR PHASE

Whether you are on BCPs or even pregnant, your egg count gradually but continually declines by approximately 5 percent per year. Every month, hundreds of immature eggs are naturally stimulated by your brain's FSH signals to be the one selected to ovulate. Only one eventually becomes the "chosen egg" and the rest become absorbed by your body.

As your endometrial lining is shedding, your body is already preparing for another attempt at pregnancy. This next part of your menstrual cycle is driven by the brain's pituitary gland production of FSH that begins to rise prior to your period. FSH was being suppressed by your ovarian hormones, but due to the drop in those hormones, FSH rises and peaks around cycle days two, three, and four. From FSH stimulating ovarian follicles, one of the follicles becomes dominant, grows, and ultimately releases the egg at ovulation. Once the dominant follicle has been selected, its estradiol (estrogen) production lowers FSH.

The first half of your cycle is dominated by the ovarian hormone estradiol that is stimulated by FSH and produced by the supporting cells of each of your eggs. Estradiol causes thickening of the uterine lining (endometrium), which prepares it to receive a fertilized egg.

MIDCYCLE—THE OVULATORY PHASE

When estradiol levels are adequately high and the dominant follicle is between 18 to 25 millimeters (0.1 to 1 inch) by averaging length and width, these two events trigger the pituitary gland to releases a surge of LH, marking the beginning of the Ovulatory Phase. This LH surge is critical for human reproduction and remains elevated for 50 hours in order to

1. Break down the ovarian cyst wall to release the egg (ovulation)
2. Increase the production of progesterone (to prepare the uterine lining for embryo implantation)
3. Mature the egg to allow fertilization (by stimulating completion of a biological process called meiosis)

FAST FACT: This LH surge is the basis of the common OPK you purchase at a pharmacy. At ovulation, high levels of LH can be detected in your urine, which turns the kit "positive," thereby signaling impending ovulation. (Of note, women with PCOS often experience a false positive OPK because their LH levels remain high throughout the month as compared to ovulating women.)

THE SECOND HALF—THE LUTEAL PHASE

The follicle from which the egg was released is called the corpus luteum, and it will release progesterone, from LH signals, that helps thicken and prepare the uterine lining for implantation. The corpus luteum will produce progesterone for about eight to ten days (the luteal phase of your cycle) but will begin to resorb unless it is "rescued" by signals from the hormone of pregnancy (hCG) to continue progesterone production for a developing pregnancy until the placenta takes over progesterone production at about eight to nine weeks of pregnancy.

As early as one week after fertilization, you can begin looking for pregnancy symptoms. You can also begin testing for pregnancy as early as 7 to 10 days past your ovulation date with an early detection urine pregnancy test (UPT). If fertilization does not occur, the egg dissolves after 24 hours. As a result, your hormone levels will decrease and your uterine lining will begin to shed about 12 to 16 days from ovulation. This is menstruation and brings us back to day one of your cycle.

The orchestration then begins all over again.

FAST FACTS—DID YOU KNOW?

The timing of ovulation is one of the most important things you should understand about your body since it is the determining factor in getting pregnant and/or preventing a pregnancy.

- Menstrual cycle intervals but are typically 28 to 30 days long, but can vary
- The Follicular Phase has the most variation and is generally between 12 and 16 days in length.
- The Luteal Phase is a more programmed 12 to 14 days. Very irregular cycles or cycles that are longer than 35 days are frequently without ovulation.

In Conclusion

Your best times to conceive are the three days surrounding ovulation, best determined by an over-the-counter OPK to detect your urine LH surge, namely, from the day before, the day of, and the day after your LH surge.

CHAPTER 5

The Reality of Ovarian Age Testing

" **Y**ou're not that good of a salesman," is what the patient declared following my nearly one-hour consultation. Confused, I asked the reasoning for her statement. "Because we came here for surrogacy and you are also discussing the alternative of adoption. I'm sure that's not good for your business if we go to an adoption agency." The words, "not good for your business," lingered in my mind with discomfort and disdain. While every medical practice must meet its financial obligations, the day a physician counsels a patient by considering the financial gain to his/her medical practice, he or she ethically and philosophically leaves medicine. Once the best interest of the patient competes with the best interest of the business, the oath of medicine becomes moot.

In practice for over 20 years, I empower my patients through extensive education of their problem and instill control back in their lives by allowing them to participate in the treatment decision. My goal is to alleviate the burden of your journey, promptly. Providing all options of family building at the initial visit, I attempt to alleviate stress, dispel myths, and explore the potential fulfillment of approaches that you may not have considered and/or avoided from prior misinformation.

The approach to overcoming infertility involves a physical, emotional, and financial investment. My obligation is to bear all these factors in mind when providing counsel. Particularly with infertility, treatment options are far from guaranteed and carry significant price tags due to the lack of nationally mandated insurance coverage. And, while adopting a child through a private agency is not inexpensive, the process of IVF surrogacy (using IVF to create embryos that will be transferred into a surrogate) often exceeds the cost of adoption.

Patients may struggle while choosing between surrogacy and adoption, but they are equally challenged when confronted with the options of adoption vs. egg donation, often stemming from the woman's DOR. Among all the pitfalls of infertility screening methods, ovarian age testing for DOR is probably the most imprecise and the most difficult for physicians to explain the implications to patients. Ultimately, patients want to know their chance for conception if their ovarian age testing is poor.

Ovarian Aging and Fighting Nature

As more women are delaying childbirth, their surge in advancing reproductive age brings the increasing problem of ovarian aging, namely, DOR. Regarding fertility and DOR, determining the quantity and quality of eggs is of great importance in providing realistic expectations to a woman for a chance of a successful pregnancy. As I explained in my **SWAT** analysis from chapter 2, DOR may result in impaired fertilization of the egg, reduced implantation, and increased miscarriages due to chromosomal abnormalities of the embryo.

Let's go further into understanding this concept by reviewing basic biology. For a woman, you are born with your entire lifetime endowment of oocytes (eggs), approximately one to two million, reduced from six to seven million while you were a 20-week fetus. Of all your eggs, approximately 1 percent eventually undergo ovulation. At the time of first menses at puberty, called menarche, your egg number has diminished to approximately 300,000 to 400,000. Each menstrual cycle is the result of several months of hundreds of eggs preparing to mature; only one (rarely two) achieves ovulation each month, while the remaining eggs become absorbed by the body. This contrasts with men, for whom spermatogenesis (sperm production) begins at puberty and continues throughout their lifetime. (For additional information on this, please see chapter 8: Optimizing Men's Prenatal Health.)

For women, no matter how you feel or look, how long you were on BCPs, or how old your mother or grandmother was when she had her last child, your ovaries will age and your pregnancy rate will be based on your birthday—that's it. Your peak fertility occurs before age 30 and after that—GULP—it's uphill. The monthly fecundity rate (ability to conceive) for ages 20 to 30 is approximately 20 percent, then declines to less than 10 percent at age 35, dropping to 5 percent at age 40, and keeps dropping thereafter. Miscarriages increase inversely as women age: 10 percent at age less than 30 to one-third of pregnancies at age 40 and they keep increasing as you age.

Comparing the Tests—the Holy Grail

Ah, but if only we could provide women the ultimate test for fertility. Some clinics and biotech companies advertise they do, forcing women into fertility doctors' offices to find out "if they are fertile," "what's the quality of my eggs," or "how many eggs do I have left." So do we have the answers to these questions? I reply with a resounding, "No" that leaves patients with more frustration and confusion.

Several markers have been used to measure ovarian age, but the most popular ones are blood tests for FSH and AMH. We have already talked about AMH and AFC in my **SWAT** analysis; see page 18. The FSH blood test is the oldest ovarian age test and should be obtained on menstrual cycle days two, three, or four. FSH has been the gold standard, but it is an indirect measurement because its level is based on feedback from hormones produced by the ovary, namely estrogen (called estradiol). Since they can fluctuate monthly, FSH testing is highly variable and valuable only if the level is elevated. Ultimately, unless the level is elevated, an FSH in the normal range is virtually meaningless for ovarian age testing.

Lastly, the fertility medication, clomiphene citrate (Clomid or CC) has also been used to measure a women's ovarian age. How does it work? The clomiphene citrate challenge test (CCCT) uses the common fertility drug to trick the brain and see how it responds to thinking the ovaries are running out of gas (low estrogen). The result? The brain's pituitary releases the hormone FSH to increase stimulation to the ovary. The higher the FSH on menstrual day 3 or 10 and after taking 100mg of CC a day from days 5 to 9, the more likely a woman has significant ovarian age. Does it work? It's certainly a helpful test, but it is time-consuming by wasting a woman's entire menstrual cycle and it's outdated.

TO AN INFERTILE WOMAN, A ONE-MONTH DELAY IN TTC FEELS LIKE ONE YEAR.

The CCCT is rarely, if ever, used because for more than 10 years, an AMH blood level has become the gold standard of ovarian age testing. All these ovarian age tests help reproductive specialists only to know the dose of injectable fertility medications to prescribe to women to stimulate her ovary to produce multiple eggs.

The Holy Grail test of ovarian aging to accurately predict your chance for fertility and/or menopause does not yet exist. Advanced maternal age (AMA) results in declining egg quality, while elevations in FSH or low AMH reflects decreasing egg numbers. In the competition between quality vs. quantity, I choose quality every time, that is, you would rather be younger with fewer eggs than older with an above average egg count. Remember, as I keep repeating, your age is the most important factor to define your fertility, not ovarian age tests. To best avoid the potential pitfalls of screening methods, it is important to remember the best screening method is to determine a women's biologic ovarian age, chronologic age, AMH level, and the number of small (< 10 mm [< 0.4 in.]) cysts, measured by ultrasound, on the ovaries (AFC).

Case Study: Ovarian Aging

The couple had already adopted two children several years earlier; yet, as the patient approached 43 years of age, she longed for one more attempt at childbearing. After many fertility specialists told her she could not succeed, she came to me for a consultation. In addition to her advanced reproductive age, her challenges included a congenital absence of her left ovary and half of her uterus (unicornuate uterus), multiple uterine leiomyomata, and her husband's severely low sperm count.

Despite such a long list of challenges, she realized her dream when she delivered a healthy daughter after IVF. (At the age of 43, she was the oldest patient I had successfully assisted—until a few years later when a 46-year-old patient of mine became the oldest woman in the United States to deliver a baby using her own eggs through IVF.) Two years later, at the age of 45, she returned to add another child to her family. Refusing to yield to her biologic ovarian aging, she experienced several unsuccessful IVF attempts.

Not interested in egg donation, she began a final IVF cycle at the age 46. From the start of the cycle, she experienced her best response to medication, while her husband uncharacteristically demonstrated a normal sperm count. When her pregnancy test results were positive, we were all overjoyed.

During the first several weeks of pregnancy, her hormone levels appeared consistent with normal progress. However, at an estimated gestational age (EGA) of seven weeks, an ultrasound showed that her embryo's growth lagged by several weeks and did not show signs of being viable. In other words, she miscarried.

Truly devastated, this loving couple elected to resolve the pregnancy through a procedure called a dilation and curettage (D&C). During the days preceding the D&C, the patient was very anxious, calling our office repeatedly to ask why she had miscarried. She finally requested a genetic analysis of the embryo to determine the cause. On the morning of the procedure, she seemed to be at peace with her pregnancy loss.

I met the patient in the preoperative area and immediately felt her pain. She held my hand and gestured for all the other personnel to leave. She was shaking and crying. All I could do was continue to hold her hand and listen with empathy. I finally excused myself in order to bring her husband into the area while I prepared for the procedure. Although her uterus was abnormally large due to fibroid tumors, the surgery proceeded without difficulty. As usual, I visited her immediately afterward to assess her pain. I approached her stretcher and placed my hands on the guardrail. Without speaking, she slowly bent to kiss my right hand—the same hand that had just removed her "dream" child from her uterus.

I recall that day regularly, particularly when times become hectic or troubling. The couple has moved on with their lives. Ironically, as I assisted them in healing, they showed me that success is not always measured in good outcomes. They reminded me of my ultimate purpose—to relieve suffering.

And so, in response to, "You're not that good of a salesman," I say, "Thank you, and I hope I never become one."

In Conclusion

Ovarian age testing is probably the most confusing concept for both patients to understand and for physicians to explain. Please remember, testing does not predict your ability to naturally conceive. AMH and AFC are the most valuable to guide your fertility specialist on the dose of injectable medication to prescribe and to predict, approximately, the number of eggs we can expect to retrieve for egg freezing or IVF.

CHAPTER 6

Optimizing Men's Prenatal Health

Ever since I was in training for my specialty, if I asked a man what percentage represents the odds that he is the cause of infertility, he would invariably say, "10 to 20 percent." But, when I asked his female partner, she would say, "I think it's half and half." These differences of opinion quickly transform into reality check as I share the incidence of causes is roughly equal: 40 percent each with the remaining 20 percent unexplained.

Why the different answers you ask? One word—fear. Whereas half of you, namely, women, are usually desperate to find a female problem so it can be addressed. The other half of you, men, are often praying I do not find any male abnormality. When I do, a large percentage of my male patients show definitive emotions such as anger, disconnect, worry, and worst of all, shame. I have learned that the sexes display different reactions: Women need to talk about their diagnosis, but men are introspective. Both care deeply, but it affects you in unique ways.

Let's get back to the shame issue. This is a powerful emotion that can affect your emotional well-being, relationship with your partner, and sexual function. Numbers are important to men, so suboptimal numbers on the sperm analysis result in self-blame and feelings of failure.

Years ago, approaches to treating infertility were almost entirely about female causes—is she ovulating, are her tubes open, is she too old? Other than a sperm analysis, the male evaluation was extremely limited. Fast forward to the 21st century and men must realize you are literally half the issue.

The sperm analysis is a vital part of the evaluation, but it is not very predictive of fertility and we must not neglect men's health, lifestyle, environmental exposures, and age.

Health

Male reproductive health has been inversely associated with the child's increased risk of disease later in life, that is, the more severe the male-factor infertility, the higher risk of disease in the offspring. As a result, men with azoospermia (no sperm in the ejaculated semen) are at highest risk for a child's health problems.

Recent data have shown that male obesity also impairs the child's metabolic and reproductive health—suggesting that paternal health issues are transmitted to the next generation with the culprit mostly likely being the sperm. And, there is now emerging evidence that male obesity impacts negatively on male reproductive potential—not only reducing sperm count and motility but also testosterone. These men have altered physical and molecular structure of their presperm cells and ultimately mature sperm. Men who are obese have higher rates of erectile dysfunction and lower frequencies of intercourse. Fortunately there is evidence that weight reduction can correct this hormonal imbalance. It's clear that men with obesity have higher rates of infertility.

Lifestyle

Without hesitation, if you are trying to maintain optimal fertility (and health), then you should eliminate excess alcohol use and any tobacco use. Too much alcohol reduces testosterone production, risks impotence, and decreases sperm production. Cigarette smoking and alcohol both have been shown to reduce semen quality, fertilization, and embryo development to the blastocyst stage. Of note, however, current evidence does not definitively prove that smoking decreases male fertility. Prior studies have suggested marijuana negatively affects sperm quality and sperm count, but there is no evidence that shows marijuana causes birth defects. The consensus among fertility studies is that marijuana probably reduces fertility.

Competitive or athletic bicycling can cause a lot of genital friction and jostling, which increases the temperature of men's testicles. There is evidence that endurance cycling, as opposed to leisurely cycling, appears to be associated with lower sperm concentrations and a significant decrease in the percentages of normal-shaped sperm. If you bicycle five or more hours per week, your semen analysis (SA) is likely to show lower sperm concentrations and lower percentages of total motile sperm than your non-exercising counterparts. If you are TTC, I would reduce the intense bicycling to fewer than five hours per week.

Some other physical activities, such as weightlifting and outdoors work, have been associated with higher sperm concentrations, but not with greater reproductive success. And, certain sports (such as football, basketball, handball, and volleyball) were linked to an increased prevalence and severity of varicocele (increase of veins in the scrotum), offering a potential link to male infertility. My advice is a reduction in intensity of these sports while trying to have a baby. While there is no definite duration of exercise, a reasonable guide is the American Heart Association's recommends of 30 minutes of aerobic activity for five days per week. (For more on varicocele and their impairment on fertility, see chapter 14: The Male Factor.)

Environment

Keep your testicles cool! Men using saunas, hot tubs, Jacuzzis, heated car seats, and laptops (on their laps) have high testicular temperature, which can negatively impact sperm production. Radio frequency electromagnetic waves from cell phones and laptops have also been shown to have harmful effects on sperm viability and motility. However, studies have not yet demonstrated that the use of these devices has decreased the ability to father a child.

If you actively use your mobile phone (and who doesn't), your sperm may have decreased numbers, decreased motility (particularly rapid progressive motility), abnormal shapes (morphology), and decreased viability. Accordingly, these abnormalities seem to worsen with the duration of mobile phone use.

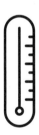

Medications

Calcium-channel blockers used for hypertension have been shown to increase cholesterol binding in the sperm head and reduce fertilization. (For a while, this medication was being studied for the potential use as a male contraceptive pill.)

Other medications that impair semen volume or sperm parameters (most of which are reversible depending on the duration of exposure) are

1. Testosterone or anabolic steroids suppress stimulating signals from the brain to the testes for sperm production and natural testosterone.
2. Opiates (narcotics) disrupt the signals that control testosterone production, which can cause low testosterone and decrease the quantity and quality of the sperm.
3. 5-alpha-reductase inhibitors (finasteride, dutasteride, and Propecia): These medications treat prostate enlargement and hair loss but also decrease sperm production.
4. Chemotherapy can reduce or stop sperm production.
5. Also of concern, the following medications may cause male fertility problems: some antibiotics, spironolactone, cimetidine, nifedipine, sulfasalazine, and colchicine.

Note: If you are TTC and you are taking one of these medications, please consult with your physician about potentially switching to an alternative effective medication that may not impair your fertility. I must stress for you not to discontinue medication unless you have been directed by your physician.

Age

While there is no clinical consensus as is the case for women, a reasonable definition of advanced paternal age is greater than 40 to 45 years. Studies have consistently reported that increasing male age is associated with an increased time to pregnancy and decreased pregnancy rates. Increasing paternal age is associated with changes in sperm DNA integrity, genetic variations (mutations) that can impact chromosomes structure and increase the risk of genetic diseases in the offspring. The risk of embryo chromosomal abnormalities does increase as men age but not to the known degree or at the same dramatic rate seen with increasing maternal age.

Advanced paternal age is associated with declining fertility and increasing miscarriages as well as increased risks of preterm births, and offspring with birth defects, autism, and schizophrenia.

Currently, there is no evidence to suggest an age above which you should not biologically procreate. However, given the increasing evidence, you may want to consider these risks in your family planning and/or look into freezing your sperm while you are in your 20s and 30s.

In Conclusion

As half the contributor to infertility, men desiring a child need to understand their lifestyle and health have significant effects on reproduction. We are also learning more about the declining fertility of the aging male. Both partners have the important responsibility to be aware of these factors in order to optimize the health of the pregnancy and baby.

CHAPTER 7

Confronting Infertility

Once you protect your fertility, you also need to know how to maximize it as well as to define infertility. In 2009 the World Health Organization (WHO) and the International Committee for Monitoring Assisted Reproductive Technologies defined infertility as "a disease of the reproductive system defined by the failure to achieve a clinical pregnancy after 12 months or more of regular unprotected sexual intercourse."

Although we strive to experience life with good health, a loving partner, a successful career, and so on, we can easily become preoccupied with our innate desire for a baby. When nature steps in and we instinctively attempt to procreate, we may also be confronted a self-proclaimed "sub-fertility," the feeling you are taking too long to conceive. It is, at these times, when a purpose can become an obsession. Sometimes, this preoccupation can be paralyzing.

But how does this type of obsession develop? And why does it often consume you, while simultaneously compelling you into stagnation?

Each of you approaches the process of building your family for unique and personal reasons. For some of you, the reasons are love of your partner and a desire to have a child created by them to share in life together. Others may fear mortality and the loss of their lineage. Women may also have the unique biologic urgency to procreate—however complicated it might be for some men to understand. Nevertheless, if a woman feels any or all these reasons, then the prospect of infertility is often the first and possibly greatest life crisis. Akin, but in some ways worse than cancer or a chronic pain syndrome, infertility has no cure—save for holding a child.

Even with the loving support of a partner, women perceive infertility as a failure in biologic, sexual, and social terms. Never can there be a moment that a childless woman is not reminded of her void through intrusive family inquiries (especially during holidays), friends' invitations to baby birthdays and showers (been there, done that), and the social script portrayed in media—in other words, when you are TTC, the world looks pregnant.

Often, women report their dreams being invaded by their longing for a child. Some cultures around the world place such an importance on childbearing that it may be accepted for a man to leave his wife in order to seek a "more fertile partner." While I have witnessed this cultural extremism, I have also observed a wide range of male emotions, from discontent to devastation and from apathy to anger, sometimes expressed for the first time in front of his partner. While a man's disconnect is worrisome for the stability of a couple's relationship, his breakthrough honesty of feelings is often therapeutic by allowing the couple to realize the impact their disease is having on each other. Lastly the inability to procreate can affect sexual identification and confidence. Unfortunately this can show up by decreasing amounts of intimacy and by performance anxiety.

Following enough frustration and worry, the couple begins the repetition and inconvenience of fertility testing and treatment. Women, although anxious, welcome the invasiveness of diagnostic probing. On the contrary, men can be so private they withdraw from visits and from physician recommendations. For the minority, months pass into years of waiting for a positive pregnancy test. The agonizing monthly menses become commonplace, and a paradoxical indifference and fear of more aggressive options and alternatives can result.

This Is When Time Clearly Halts

How we overcome adversity is a measure of our integrity and character. Our motivation to turn "lemons into lemonade" represents optimism and perseverance. The specific challenge that fertility patients endure results from mourning a life that has not been realized. I describe fertility patients as having their faces pressed "up against the windows" of families while longing to embrace the dream they do not own. Achievement of their goal may require a new perspective, one that was not originally planned.

For more than ten years, I had the unique perspective of being a fertility patient while practicing as a fertility specialist. My passion for the fertility field came first during medical school and was only intensified by my personal struggles. Through years of fertility treatments, my wife and I finally came to closure by adopting our angels. I have consequently grown more fervent in assisting others to build their family and prevent them from becoming consumed in despair. Realizing there are many ways to establish a family, patients have gained hope through the openness of my own challenge.

Seeing firsthand how infertile couples become devastated and overwhelmed, I have always firmly believed fertility is a physical, emotional, and financial investment. While the first and third of these commitments are clearly vital, many times the emotional and spiritual aspects of a patient's challenge are neglected. The importance of this contribution is demonstrated by medical studies on higher fertility rates in women with lower anxiety and depressive symptoms. As a result, my practice incorporates a full-time reproductive health psychologist. The reason for this is that the quality of life for the patient is approached in a positive and healthy way.

While there is no definitive evidence supporting the hypothesis that stress reduces fertility, medical studies using counseling appear to increase pregnancy rates. Unfortunately, because reproduction is so complicated, all the variables involved prevent a clear and concise cause and effect when considering the role of stress. To make matters worse, arguably every fertility patient has been on the receiving end of the unfounded suggestion, "Just relax and then you will get pregnant."

Why this is so devastating to the woman experiencing difficulty TTC is the self-inflicted blame-game (that her stress is preventing her from realizing her dream). While we do not know the degree stress may impact fertility, we are certain that infertility is responsible for an infertile couple's stress. Infertility clinics should be proactive in educating you on options for coping and stress reduction along your journey. The ASRM has a Mental Health Professional Group (MHPG) that promotes the "scientific understanding of the psychological, social, and emotional perspectives of infertility patients." You can find valuable resources online to guide you along your journey, as well as a directory of mental health providers who specialize in infertility. Visit connect.asrm.org/mhpg for more information.

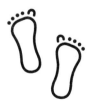

How to Get Through the Holidays

This can be especially true during the holidays, which can be trying even under the best of circumstances. Infertile couples often experience more of a challenge by fluctuating between various degrees of anger and depression, and the holiday season seems to only emphasize their sense of loss. Important first steps (anytime, but especially during the holidays) for couples to cope are recognition that these moods are common and acceptance of these emotions without guilt. Whether through professional counseling or support groups, couples can have their feelings validated, which helps them plan for the holidays with a more positive mental health.

A common "side effect" of infertility is experiencing a sense of being "out of control." As a result, preparing for the holidays can be very helpful. For example, shopping for gifts early in the season, or online, can avoid being exposed to seasonal festivities in malls and help eliminate the general stress of last-minute shopping. Three other helpful coping measures are

(1) Deciding in advance which events are comfortable for you to attend
(2) Taking a vacation or planning an elegant evening with child-free friends
(3) Responding to insensitive comments with honesty, avoidance, or even humor

As an additional measure (in case you encounter a situation in which you feel overwhelmed), have someone available you can call for support or try diverting your attention to a positive image.

Talking to an infertility specialist can provide you with answers to difficult questions—and with a plan of treatment that may give you hope and direction. An integral part of your treatment is finding a doctor who is sensitive, caring, and one in whom you have confidence. The strength that sustains couples through the diagnosis of infertility will support them through other trying times in life. Often, the couple emerges with a deeper understanding of their lives and love for each other.

Aspects of Coping

COPING WITH FAMILY AND FRIENDS . . .

A good strategy is to plan the topics you want to keep private, which subjects you are willing to discuss, and with whom. The following questions will help guide your thinking.

1. If your struggles with fertility were to last for many months or longer, who are the people that you would like to have in your support network?
2. Who should be privy to information regarding your diagnosis and treatment?
3. Who might best be left out of the information loop?
4. Bearing in mind that once information is disclosed, it cannot be restricted, how much and what kind of information is appropriate to share?
5. What types of support do you have in place to cope with anticipated and unanticipated reactions to disclosure?

INDIVIDUAL COPING STRATEGIES

To help reduce stress on a regular basis, try to engage in activities that are relaxing, provide relief, and are easy to access. Activities might include meditation, yoga, creative visualization, listening to music, deep breathing and progressive muscle relaxation techniques, hitting golf balls, or taking walks. Give yourself "little pleasures" and never forget the following:

1. Avoid exhaustion, loss of sleep, and overwork.
2. Eat regular, nourishing meals.
3. Know your limits and pace yourself accordingly.
4. Strive to develop mindfulness: Appreciate the moment, maintain a here-and-now focus, increase awareness of sights, smells, sounds, and touch in the moment.
5. Become an active participant instead of a passive recipient when managing fertility and holiday stressors.
6. Give yourself permission to be. Give yourself breathing space and expect fluctuation in your mood and perspective. Allow yourself the privilege of "limping" until wounds have healed and you can learn to run again.

COPING STRATEGIES FOR COUPLES

You and your partner will have your own individual coping strategies; however, each of you will also need to work together to decrease the stress you experience as a couple. This stress-reduction checklist for couples can help.

1. Maintain open, honest communication.
2. Plan intimate (non-sexual) time.
3. Be willing to take a break from the day-to-day "shadow" of fertility. Limit your conversation about fertility treatment to a small amount of time, maybe 30 minutes a day.
4. Develop a shared ritual, symbolic ceremony, or sign that recognizes your experiences with fertility such as planting a commemorative tree, hanging a memorial plaque, saying a prayer, and writing your deepest thoughts on dissolvable paper and placing it in water.
5. Set reasonable goals together to make social/holiday times happier and easier to manage.
6. Participate in a support group, either in your community or online.
7. Work to arrive at an emotional consensus that respects each partner's needs.
8. Respect your differences in coping strategies.
9. Struggles with fertility create difficult and stressful enough times for you and your partner—and, when combined with social/holiday settings, those stress levels can be compounded. Planning ahead can help reduce social/holiday stressors (see Coping with Family and Friends at the beginning of this section).
10. Keep in mind that you should seek professional help—either individually and/or as a couple—from a psychologist or counselor who specializes in reproductive health concerns if stress-related symptoms increase.

The Ackerman Institute Infertility Project

The inability to conceive or maintain a pregnancy frequently creates a complex developmental crisis as patients move through a series of emotional phases.

This process, similar to models used to describe coping with grief, is fluid and repetitive, not necessarily progressive or linear in form. The model developed by the staff of the Ackerman Institute for their infertility project, consists of five distinct phases that represent transitions and helps provide a framework for understanding the stress that people with infertility experience.

The *Dawning Phase* occurs as persons become increasingly aware they may have problems with conception. Then, when couples initiate medical diagnostic testing, they have moved into the *Mobilization Phase*, where there is concern about the possibility of infertility and increasing recognition of a problem. Next is the *Immersion Phase*, which is the most complicated and intense phase. At this point, there is additional medical testing and treatment—and continual uncertainty. Often, this is a period of considerable emotional turmoil, as invasive medical treatments are initiated and anticipatory grief about the possibility of childlessness emerges and grows.

The following *Resolution Phase* is marked by three subphases: (1) ending medical treatment; (2) recognizing and mourning the loss of not having a biologically related child; and (3) changing focus to other options, such as adoption. Finally, the *Legacy Phase* addresses the totality and the after-effects of an infertility struggle. At any phase of this process, psychological problems may result when struggles have not been managed effectively.

Psychological Influences

The psychological influences of infertility are a powerful and formidable factor. Sexual intimacy is often reduced to a scheduled exercise fraught with stress and anxiety about failing to conceive. In addition to the stress caused by infertility, there may be decreased sexual pleasure and desire as result of the pressure to conceive. Sexual problems and dysfunctions may arise due to the need to perform on demand. In addition, partners may feel shame, doubt, and anger with their bodies or disappointment and frustration with their partner's inability to fulfill their desire for a child.

Depressive feelings, anxiety, decreased self-esteem, shame, helplessness, and guilt are all emotional issues of infertility. Feelings of isolation, spiritual and relational abandonment, and disconnection are also problems that individuals and couples describe. It is often difficult for someone to step back and evaluate the considerable effect that infertility is having on their lives. Instead, distress becomes magnified as awareness of the infertility problem becomes undeniable, and definitions and perceptions of oneself are examined through the lens of infertility.

At this time, it is important to recognize and utilize your strengths to limit the negative experience of this problem. With the aid of therapy, the experience of infertility may help you develop strengths—such as improving communication, enhancing assertiveness, strengthening effective conflict resolution, and increasing empathy for others.

Psychologists can aid patients in moving away from this manner of self-definition and shift to the active position of, "I am struggling with infertility." People faced with infertility endure repeated "invisible losses" from unsuccessful pregnancy attempts. Therapeutic support from psychologists who specialize in reproductive health, while working in tandem with physicians, often helps patients to normalize and externalize this difficult experience.

In Conclusion

Are there other advantages to stress reduction? Often, infertility has no immediate cure. The diagnosis begins a journey that can be arduous. The road toward any goal has the potential to be as rewarding and inspiring (if not more so) as the destination.

Obviously, one cannot argue the extreme fulfillment of finally holding your new baby. Yet, along this challenging path, unrealistic expectations may surface as well as a dramatic enlightenment about ourselves as we endure with newfound strength, direction, and inner peace. All this may allow for a spiritual awakening, while on the surface it appears to be your darkest hour.

My personal credo has always been, "The people who face stress and remain healthy, thus perceive change not as a threat but as a challenge and sense of opportunity." It has and will always be my privilege to be involved in this aspect of your lives, and I gain inspiration from watching how you all confront and overcome your struggles.

CHAPTER 8

Confronting Secondary Infertility

When you have one child but are having difficulty conceiving another, this is called *secondary infertility*—inability to conceive after six months of attempts and no risk factors. Unlike primary infertility (when a couple has never experienced a pregnancy after at least one year of attempting to do so through unprotected intercourse), there are no accurate statistics on the number of women and couples facing secondary infertility.

Do you feel the same disappointment, frustration, and void from primary infertility as you do with secondary? The following seven points explain the difference.

1. No One Validates You

People often frustrate women facing secondary infertility with the advice, "you should feel blessed having had a child and be grateful for their miracle since other women struggle to have their first child." Unfortunately these comments to those of you with secondary infertility are emotionally damaging because they can almost make you feel guilty for desiring to grow your family. Simply put, no person's advice can fully relieve or comfort you when you are challenged with infertility. Each of your support people needs to recognize that infertility is devastating, whether it is for a first or subsequent child.

Bottom Line: Your friends and family need to know that anytime a woman is having trouble conceiving, a sensitive and supportive approach is crucial to validating her challenge.

2. This Time It's for Your Child

When you decide to have a first child, you are often seeking personal and relationship fulfillment, the creation of a family, along with the joy of bringing life into the world and rearing your child.

Primary infertility disrupts your life's plan and can cause powerful feelings, which include inadequacy, vulnerability, and a sense of being overwhelmed, as well as the potential disruption of your relationship. Once there is an existing child, the decision to grow your family, in addition to the above reasons, often stems from a profound and selfless desire to provide your one child a sibling with whom to share their life and develop a history.

Consequently, while a woman's or couple's disappointment from primary infertility originates from their intrinsic desires, secondary infertility often stems from the needs of the existing child. Did you ever hear your parents tell you that they love you more than themselves? Secondary infertility is devastating since it deprives and disappoints their existing child.

Bottom Line: The desire for a second child as a sibling can be equally if not more compelling than for the initial child.

3. Usually Explainable

While 20 percent of primary infertility is considered unexplainable, the percentage of unexplained secondary cases is much lower, though no actual statistic is agreed upon. Secondary infertility is usually due to something having changed since the prior conception, which is now resulting in infertility.

Examples of such a "change" include advancing age (usually the female—but more evidence is accumulating on the male partner), tubal ligation, pelvic surgery with resultant scarring, female and/or male significant weight gain, partner vasectomy, and more rarely, uterine scarring following D&C for miscarriage and the subsequent development of an isthmocele (a chronic fluid collection inside the uterus at the site of the scar following a cesarean section).

Bottom Line: The good news is that when a cause is discovered, treatment can be directed at the problem area for an improved chance of pregnancy.

4. Doctor Delays a.k.a. Dragging Their Feet

As a fertility specialist, I have rarely seen one of you who did not want to have a baby yesterday. By the time you get to see me, you are usually spent. Here is your typical path, depending on your age: 6 to 12 months of TTC; 6 to 12 months with your OB/GYN, sitting in their reception area with all pregnant women ("oh what joy!") and being tested, checking your blood for ovulation, your tubes with a hysterosalpingogram (HSG), and your partner's sperm sample, and then given clomiphene citrate or other fertility medication. After all this, plus internet surfing and self-diagnosing and still no BOB (baby on board), you or your partner, mother, best friend, or hopefully OB/GYN office recommends a fertility specialist. At which time, I repeat, you are spent!

Since you already have a child, your doctor may delay in referring you to a fertility specialist because he/she presumes you will readily conceive again. "Don't worry, it will happen just like last time," are words patients share from their physicians, family, and friends. However, when you feel there is a problem, we as fertility specialists need to address those concerns to reduce your stress, shatter myths, and direct you quickly toward evidence-based treatment.

And I'm not laying unfounded claims as a marketing tool to see fertility specialists right away. Studies have shown that pregnancy is achieved in a shorter time period when you are promptly referred. In delaying the referral, your increasing frustration can prolong your time to pregnancy and make it less likely for you to return to your original OB/GYN for pregnancy care once your fertility specialists assist you.

Bottom Line: With secondary infertility, you should see a fertility specialist if you are under the age of 35 and have been TTC for 6 to 12 months; age 35 to 39 and have been TTC for three to six months; over the age of 39 and unable to conceive no longer than three months; or sooner for all scenarios if you are without regular periods and/or if there are risk factors of concern.

5. Age

My patients, regardless of their gender, never like to talk about their age. During consultations with my female patients, they invariably advance their age, sometimes by years! For example, a 27-year-old will express her anxiety over infertility by saying, "You know Dr. T, I'm not getting any younger and 30 is right around the corner" to which I reply, "you'll have to walk that street for three years before you reach it." Other patients in their early 30s picture themselves as practically 35 already, and 35-year-olds often imagine they are effectively 40.

Whether or not you had difficulty conceiving your first child, age will always enter the factor when TTC your second or additional children. In other words, whether you experienced primary infertility or not, age, both for the woman and man, will play a role in reducing fertility. There is simply no escaping the biological clock.

The greatest indicator of fertility is a woman's age. Your peak fertility occurs up until age 30. Subsequently and gradually, as a women and men age, fertility declines and miscarriages increase (mostly due to chromosomal abnormalities of the aging egg). If you had prior infertility, you may be more aggressive seeking treatment sooner. But, without a history of infertility, you may prolong TTC naturally or by using conservative treatment.

Bottom Line: Be aggressive with your fertility if you are above age 35, and consider proceeding directly to IVF if you are above age 39.

6. Your First Pregnancy (After Stopping the Pill) Was Easy

A funny thing happens after taking the birth control pill (BCP) for years due to irregular periods—it has a high chance to restore your period, briefly. Why? We are not certain but the condition of PCOS seems to respond to the hormone regulation of the BCP resulting in temporary ovulation cycles. The result? Improved fertility right after stopping the BCP.

Becoming pregnant soon after coming off the BCP, you may not realize you had PCOS (see chapter 13). When you try for a second child, this time without the BCP, you may be disappointed when you do not conceive readily. The ovulation dysfunction of PCOS was hidden while you were on BCP but normalizes for at least for the first three to six months following discontinuation.

One of the many known BCP benefits is menstrual cycle regulation, which is why it is used effectively in managing PCOS, the most common hormonal disorder of women. Women with PCOS struggle from ovulation dysfunction and unwanted hair growth along with the medical risks of weight gain, prediabetes, elevated blood pressure/cholesterol, and risk of uterine cancer.

PCOS affects up to 20 percent of all women in their reproductive years. This most common of hormonal imbalances often requires ovulation induction usually in the form of prescribed tablets. The American College of Obstetricians and Gynecologists (ACOG) recently recommended letrozole as the first-line treatment for ovulation induction in PCOS women, given the higher pregnancy rates when compared with clomiphene citrate. A minor outpatient surgery called ovarian diathermy is also very effective at restoring ovulation spontaneously. (We'll cover this further in chapter 13.)

When a woman with PCOS desires their second child, they are often either not taking BCP for enough time or never resumed postpartum; hence, their secondary infertility results from a lack of ovulation.

Bottom Line: See a fertility specialist promptly if your menstrual cycles are irregular.

7. Tubal Ligation or Vasectomy

As obvious obstructions in the ability to conceive, a woman's tubal ligation and the man's vasectomy are surgical procedures that induce secondary infertility and allow only two options for fertility—surgical reversal to open the tubes or ducts respectively, or proceeding to IVF. Contrary to prior belief, vasectomy reversal success is not based on the number of years from the original procedure. Success rates for both tubal and vasectomy reversal procedures are driven by the woman's age. As a result, younger women have the options of tubal reversal or vasectomy, but women above the age of 35 to 37 should give strong consideration for IVF.

In a man with an unreversed vasectomy, IVF also requires the retrieval of sperm through a minor procedure that removes sperm from its storage and transport area (epididymis), either by a microsurgical epididymal sperm aspiration (MESA) or directly from the testis, called testicular sperm aspiration (TESA). Sperm retrieved in this manner are not mature enough to fertilize naturally and cannot be artificially inseminated into a woman's uterus. Testicular sperm not only requires IVF but also the advanced fertilization technique of ICSI (intracytoplasmic sperm injection) to achieve fertilization of the egg. The use of MESA or TESA does appear to result in slightly lower IVF success rather than with ejaculated sperm.

Bottom Line: Tubal ligation/vasectomy options should be driven by the female partner's age, the success rate of the surgeon/clinic, as well as the cost of the procedures.

In Conclusion

Secondary infertility can be equally, if not more, frustrating than primary because fewer people validate your concerns—including, sometimes, your OB/GYN. Prompt referral to an infertility specialist has been shown to shorten the time to pregnancy. Be proactive and seek a specialist sooner rather than later, particularly if the carrying partner is above age 35.

FAST FACTS

Will You Need IVF Again?

Success with a prior IVF cycle does increase the chance for a baby if IVF is repeated. However, as with all medical procedures, there are advantages and disadvantages to having a medical procedure.

a. Advantage—Been There, Done That

Part of the anxiety a woman experiences with fertility treatment—particularly IVF—is the unknown, namely, concern over medication side effects, self-administering injections, the egg retrieval, and, ultimately, whether she will conceive. Having undergone IVF, a woman may, though not always, be more comfortable during the process the second time around.

The IVF clinic staff must always realize, despite a woman already having one or more children, she can be just as anxious, or even more so than a woman without a child, to grow her family. Whether stress reduction equates to a higher pregnancy rate is a topic of considerable debate without a definitive scientific conclusion, though the medical literature does favor the association. Nevertheless, methods to reduce stress in a woman during an IVF cycle results in an improved quality of life and is certainly a prudent goal.

b. Advantage—Higher Pregnancy Rate

You have a higher pregnancy rate with a repeat IVF cycle if you successfully had a child in a prior IVF cycle. A previously successful IVF treatment cycle also allows the physician and patient to review the prior cycle to duplicate favorable decisions that were beneficial and exclude those that did not appear valuable. While a pregnancy is not guaranteed, the statistical improvement can comfort a patient with the decision to repeat an IVF cycle.

c. Disadvantage—Expectations

The expectations for a repeat IVF cycle may be unrealistic depending upon the individual circumstances. As mentioned, success in a prior IVF cycle does not guarantee the same number of eggs retrieved, embryos developed, or a pregnancy, particularly as the length of time from the prior IVF cycle increases. This is because ovarian aging influences the number of eggs retrieved from a woman with IVF, that is, as a woman ages she continues to decrease her number of eggs due to natural biology.

CHAPTER 9

An Overview of Infertility Causes and a Guide to the First Steps in a Fertility Evaluation

While the field of reproductive medicine continues to advance treatment options, we must first diagnose your reason for infertility. As mentioned in an earlier chapter, men and women have equal percentages of causes of their infertility, that is, about 40 percent each with 20 percent unexplained and 30 percent some combination of factors.

Not only is the cause percentage divided between the sexes misunderstood by many of you, but knowing the percentage chances for a natural pregnancy is often as equal to the challenge of knowing a Final Jeopardy question! Let's give it another try—the natural peak monthly fertility rate occurs for women less than or equal to age 30 and it is 20 to 25 percent. After one year of TTC, cumulatively about 85 percent of you will be successful; 92 percent after two years, and 93 percent after three years.

Which brings me to this—you know all your girlfriends who post on social media about how fast they got pregnant? Well, I hate to break it to you and them but . . . they are probably fibbing or, at least, exaggerating! I know all about the exhilaration of posting the big news! But fair is fair. My fertility warriors who follow my Facebook medical practice page (fb.com/myfertilitycare) know it's improbable for *all* their girlfriends to get pregnant the exact month they want. It just isn't statistically likely.

Now we turn to the 35-year-old age group: Approximately 10 percent of you will get pregnant each month. Then there are the sobering numbers at age 40: Only 5 percent of you will conceive on a monthly basis.

The basic infertility evaluation has remained constant and focused on the most common areas of abnormality: 40 percent female factor—subdivided into 40 percent ovulation dysfunction and 40 percent fallopian tube blockage; 40 percent male factor; and 20 percent unexplained. Infertility affects approximately one in every eight couples and is generally accepted as the absence of a live birth after one year of attempting pregnancy in a woman with monthly menstrual cycles and no prior risk of the couple toward infertility.

Within one menstrual cycle, your infertility evaluation can be efficiently completed by performing an HSG between menstrual cycle days six through twelve, testing for presumptive ovulation by urine OPKs or appropriately-timed blood progesterone, and obtaining a comprehensive SA. Because of inconsistent insurance coverage for infertility patients, physicians must be conscious of a cost-effective, evidence-based approach to the evaluation.

Progesterone levels indicate the hormone changes consistent with ovulation. If you have monthly cycles, this test should be done about one week prior to your expected period. For example, in a typical 28-day menstrual cycle, a progesterone blood test should be obtained on approximately days 21 to 24.

Your First Visit

The anxiety and fear I see on your faces during the first visit with me is always heartbreaking. You certainly want to see I am attentive, personable, and empathic. Hopefully, you all vetted me for my qualifications prior to your visit by asking your OB/GYN and your friends about me, reading reviews, and visiting our social media sites. While I love to spend time getting to know—origins, job, hobbies—I can see in your eyes a special need.

It took me several years in practice to realize the one common fear all my patients have that manifests during their first visit. At our initial consultation and during every subsequent encounter with you, I always include one question, "How are you really doing?" This inquiry is often met with every emotion one can portray—sadness, anger, frustration, grief, denial, confusion, and distress. But, typically, during the first visit, my patients cry after I ask this profound question. Sometimes, they simply show mild tears and explain their sorrow, and other times, they need much more time to vent their frustration. Either way, it is therapeutic to express your emotion. Often, my patients tell me it's the first time a physician ever asked them about their coping ability.

As a faculty member in the University of Central Florida College of Medicine, who teaches OB/GYN residents and medical students, I emphasize the psychological aspect of this disease, "Never underestimate the devastation of infertility." No matter how you all initially appear—laughing, indifferent, even aloof—there is usually a mask waiting to be removed. I have further come to believe there is an inverse relationship between your mood during your visit and your true devastation, that is, the ones who are smiling and happy are often the same ones who are the most crushed over their infertility.

So what is this one paralyzing fear at the time of your first visit that haunts you until we address it? I learned this from my patient over ten years ago. Michelle (not her real name) was a 30-year-old with a successful job, happy marriage, and positive outlook on life. She appeared to have realistic expectations over her fertility. Yet, when we got to the money question, "How are you really doing?" she began to cry. Without exaggeration, she was tearful for almost 30 minutes. The reason—she was waiting for me to tell her she would never be a mother. Her fear was that I would discover an irreversible reason for her infertility that no medical or surgical treatment could overcome. She cried so long that she brought us several boxes of tissues at her next visit because she used up so many!

I am grateful for all my patients' openness to express their disappointment. Truth be told, I have never made the following statement, "I am sorry, but you will never be a mother (or father)." This is not because of my exceptional prowess as a physician— though I wish it were!

Rather I believe that, with advanced reproductive technology and alternative options, you all have a strong potential to be a parent, whether through using your eggs with partner sperm, egg donation, sperm donation, surrogacy, or adoption. While I understand the original goal is typically always to use your own eggs and/or sperm, I share the other options as a means of providing hope, encouragement, and support toward ultimately having a child, if you are open to all methods.

History

For me to gain insight into why you are having trouble conceiving, I acquire your complete obstetric, gynecologic, medical, surgical, and family history. As a woman, once again, your age is the single most predictive factor to gauge your ability to have a baby. Additional important factors affecting your prognosis include your years of infertility and whether you have had a prior live birth.

What can you tell about yourself? Simply looking at your menstrual cycle interval can speak volumes about your ovulation function. The best way is to use an inexpensive over-the-counter urine OPK. This is far superior to BBT charts or phone apps! BBTs are not reliable, do not predict, and only suggest recent past ovulation. They're not helpful to proactively conceive. And please don't get me started on the apps! These are calculated predictors of ovulation based on your menstrual interval history. They are not biological predictors, so forget about their relying on your cervical mucus, LH surge, and lower abdominal cramping. HINT: If your cycles are regular, then you presumably ovulate two weeks from your next first day of menses, that is, a 28-day interval ovulated on day 14, a 30-day interval ovulates on day 16, etc. There, I saved you the cost of buying an app!

How about your ovarian age? DOR can be suggested by irregular period intervals, a lessening of the duration and intensity of your menstrual cycles, along with vasomotor symptoms, such as vaginal dryness and hot flashes—a sudden onset of extreme warmth and flushness of your face and upper chest, which last seconds to minutes throughout the day and even the night.

Your period intervals and flow are extremely important as a sign of hormonal stability.

Irregular period intervals often represent a hormonal imbalance called PCOS and absent periods may also reflect PCOS (see chapter 13) as well as conditions such as eating disorders, excessive exercise (the Female Athlete Triad), pituitary tumor, or ovarian failure (primary ovarian insufficiency). Further, dysmenorrhea (painful periods) and dyspareunia (painful intercourse) can be a sign of endometriosis (normal uterine lining that implants anywhere else in the body, detailed in chapter 12, Endometriosis: Pain or Infertility?).

Other gynecologic factors that are explored in the initial evaluations:

• Coital frequency and timing, or lack thereof, with ovulation
• Erection/ejaculation/semen volume dysfunction
• Use of lubricants that may be toxic to sperm
• Prior gynecologic surgeries—involving your tubes or removal of fibroid tumors; all pelvic surgeries may cause scarring that can reduce fertility.
• Prior pelvic infections—The risks of a tubal cause of infertility are five times higher after a single episode of a pelvic infection.

Your prior medical records of diagnostic tests should be reviewed to prevent redundancy of testing and a delay in treatment.

Physical Examination

As a fertility patient, you should undergo a complete physical exam with attention to blood pressure, BMI, thyroid, and evidence of hirsutism (dark coarse adult hair growth in male pattern areas). Other important areas suggesting hormonal issues include galactorrhea (milky nipple discharge), weight changes, acne, and frontal balding. The extremes of body weight always pose reproductive challenges for women, usually by affecting ovulation function. While there are studies that question the true impact of an elevated BMI on fertility, the negative impact remains regarding an increased risk of miscarriage and higher pregnancy complications.

Over the years, reproductive medicine clinics have gradually replaced the pelvic exam with a pelvic transvaginal ultrasound (TUVS). The use of TUVS allows evaluation of the pelvis equal to, if not superior to, a pelvic exam by visualizing the ovaries for PCOS as well as for masses suggestive of endometriomas (ovarian cysts of endometriosis), and the uterus for fibroids (benign uterine tumors).

For many years, the PCT was a routine part of the physical infertility evaluation to look at viable sperm in the vagina hours after intercourse. The PCT was supposed to screen you for antisperm antibodies. But a randomized research trial comparing patients having a PCT versus not being tested revealed the former undergo additional testing with no significant difference on pregnancy outcome. It is considered outdated, so there is no strong evidence compelling you to have a PCT—I've never even performed one on a patient!

Ovarian Age Testing

(For additional information on ovarian age testing, please see chapter 6: The Reality of Ovarian Age Testing.)

It's highly likely that this is the most confusing concept for us to counsel you (i.e., the quantity and quality of your egg pool). Women are born with one to two million eggs, reduced to 300,000 to 500,000 at puberty, and then approximately 10,000 remain at age 37 while a woman ovulates from 300 to 500 follicles during her reproductive life span.

Your monthly chance for a pregnancy begins a steady decline after the female ages of 30 and the male age of 40. Some women experience DOR at an earlier age, varying from mild DOR to full-blown premature ovarian failure (POF), which is the cessation of ovarian function before the age of 40 (now called, primary ovarian insufficiency). Your age tells us about your egg quality; hormone tests and ultrasound estimates your remaining number of eggs. Blood FSH used to be the main test but, due to the monthly fluctuations, it is only a valuable tool if the result is abnormal (elevated). I consider FSH an outdated test for ovarian aging.

Over the past few years, AMH, produced by ovarian granulosa cells (supporting cells of eggs), has surpassed FSH as the more reliable and valid tool to measure DOR. Not requiring a feedback mechanism from the ovary like FSH, AMH's other distinction is the ability to be measured any day of your menstrual cycle, even while on BCPs, and it is an earlier predictor of DOR. Ultimately, a test to predict the age of menopause remains elusive.

> Prolonged BCPs can falsely and temporarily lower your AMH level. For an accurate reading, you may want to discontinue BCPs for several months prior to AMH testing.

Genetics

All of you planning a pregnancy should be offered genetic testing to determine if you carry a single-gene defect; think cystic fibrosis, sickle cell, or Tay-Sachs disease. There is ongoing debate as to which disorders should be tested, but if you are a carrier, your partner or egg/sperm donor needs to be tested, too. If both biological parents are carriers of the same gene mutation, then the baby has a 25 percent chance of inheriting a potentially fatal disease.

The two genetic disorders recommended by the American College of Obstetricians and Gynecologists (ACOG) and the American College of Medical Genetics and Genomics (ACMG) for which all women planning a pregnancy should be screened are cystic fibrosis and spinal muscular atrophy. For women with severe ovarian aging (primary ovarian insufficiency) or a family history of Fragile X or intellectual disability, then Fragile X screening is advised as well. Women of Mediterranean, Middle Eastern, Southeast Asian, or West Indian descent are advised to have testing for blood disorders called thalassemia or sickle cell, which can cause severe anemia. Screening for Tay-Sachs disease should be offered if the woman or couple are of Ashkenazi Jewish, French-Canadian, or Cajun descent.

Every human cell has 23 pairs of chromosomes, for a total of 46. A normal female is labelled 46, XX (the two X chromosomes are female); a man is labelled 46, XY (the Y is the male chromosome). Each chromosome contains hundreds to thousands of genes.

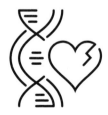

Male Infertility

As men, you have biologic testicular aging with negative consequences on fertility. Medical studies of male infertility are increasingly exploring the reproductive associations of advancing paternal age (usually considered as past the age of 40) to include declining numbers on a SA, higher miscarriage and birth defects, and autism and schizophrenia of their children. You also will have an increased risk of infertility with a history of

- Cryptorchidism (One or both testes are undescended—not in the scrotal sac—at birth; the longer they remain this way, the higher the likelihood of infertility.)
- Unilateral orchiectomy (surgical removal of a testis)
- Chemotherapy and radiation for a cancer

If your SA shows abnormalities, you should undergo a genital exam, along with hormonal testing, by a urologist trained in male infertility. So often I see men referred to my practice with an abnormal sperm analysis who have undergone advanced fertility procedures like IUI or even IVF without a prior urology exam. Why is this important? Because an abnormal sperm analysis could be your first sign of a serious disease in the testes, estimated to occur in 1 to 2 percent of men.

JUST SAY NO TO TESTOSTERONE!

Bob (not real name) is a 38-year-old accountant who has gained weight gradually over the years. He rarely exercises due to "a lack of time" and his BMI is 34 kg/m². He presented with his wife for infertility. She is 32 with regular periods, a normal HSG, blood progesterone for ovulation, and BMI. Bob shared that his primary care physician placed him on injectable testosterone twice weekly due to a "borderline" low blood testosterone level obtained because he had been complaining of gradually worsening fatigue.

I immediately said to myself two words: "Uh Oh."

First, a little background. Your testes (like the ovaries) talk to your brain and it listens very, very well. Stimulated by the pituitary, the testes produce testosterone, which feeds back to the brain. This cross talk between the testes and pituitary keeps the correct amount of hormone levels in each area. The same thing occurs with the ovaries— they tell the brain there is enough estradiol (estrogen) so the brain can lower the stimulation. It's a delicate balance between the brain and the gonads (testes or ovaries) but it works. If the brain senses enough or higher than needed testosterone, the pituitary's LH hormone signal to the testes reduces.

Unfortunately, injectable testosterone is a potent suppressant of the pituitary and can result in a complete shutdown of stimulation to the testes. You see, the brain doesn't care where testosterone originates—from the testes, a tumor, or outside the body through medicine—it just responds accordingly and reduces its signal to the testes, sometimes to minimal. The consequences of this scenario can be dire to reproduction, namely, the testes profound reduction of sperm production to the point of no sperm in the ejaculate (azoospermia). This condition of testes suppression can be reversible unless the man has been taking prolonged injectable testosterone (for at least one year).

Let's get back to Bob. Without exception, one of the most frustrating and damaging prescriptions that are given to a man in their reproductive years is testosterone. Many doctors, and patients, imagine its effects to be like the fountain of youth. Too many doctors order a blood test for testosterone for men complaining of fatigue or simply as a "routine" screen. I disagree emphatically with this approach.

Bob presented as a middle-aged man, overweight, who doesn't exercise. In the United States, unfortunately, there are too many Bobs. His physical condition is the most likely explanation for his fatigue. Bob is most likely suffering from a lack of exercise and obesity, both contributing to his fatigue. But many physicians who treat men, like Bob, feel compelled to put pen in hand and on a prescription pad—much to the damage of men's reproduction. It's also worth noting that obesity lowers testosterone levels.

As you can imagine, the sperm analysis I ordered on Bob came back as azoospermia (no sperm in the semen). He was devastated. He discontinued his testosterone and scheduled a consultation with our male reproductive urologist.

Over time Bob did not recover sperm in his semen. He underwent a testicular sperm retrieval followed by IVF-ICSI and they were successful in having a child.

Anatomical Evaluation

HSG is the gold standard screening test for a woman's fallopian tubes to determine if they are patent (open). This test involves injecting contrast dye into your cervix and uses fluoroscopy X-ray to watch the path of the dye through your uterus and fallopian tubes. We can tell if the inside of the uterus is normal or has abnormal filling of dye that will prompt further testing to confirm a suspected abnormality, for example, polyps (benign overgrowth of normal tissue); fibroids (benign uterine tumor); scar tissue (called Asherman's syndrome); or a congenital variation in the cavity shape called a mullerian anomaly (occurring during embryo development).

The HSG also provides valuable information regarding the condition of the fallopian tubes—if they are blocked and where they are blocked. When the part of the tube closest to the uterus is blocked, called proximal tubal occlusion, we cannot be sure if this is due to a true problem with the tube or due to the uterus having a temporary spasm of the tiny muscles surrounding the tube. To distinguish these causes, we can prepare for a procedure to open the tube, called a tubal cannulation, where a very thin guide wire is used to bypass the blockage. At the time of the procedure, while the woman is under sedation, we first repeat the dye injection—if the tube(s) is/are now open, the original HSG result was a false positive.

The other tubal problem is blockage furthest from the uterus and closest to the ovary, called distal tubal occlusion. This condition is often associated with a serious tubal problem that we call a hydrosalpinx (the blocked swollen end of the fallopian tube is filled with fluid). Natural fertility is impaired, even if only one tube is a hydrosalpinx and the other is normal because the tubal fluid can travel back into the uterine cavity to reduce implantation. A hydrosalpinx is most concerning if it is seen by pelvic ultrasound. A pelvic ultrasound does not visualize normal fallopian tubes. Many studies have supported surgery for tubal interruption or salpingectomy (removing a tube) to prevent the toxic fluid of the hydrosalpinx from travelling back into the uterus. I agree and have performed this surgery for many patients to improve outcome either naturally or with IVF. Studies promote best outcomes when the entire hydrosalpinx tube is removed.

Endometriosis

Simply defined, endometriosis is normal uterine lining found, at the time of surgery, anywhere else in your body than where it's supposed to be. We can confirm the diagnosis of endometriosis only by surgical biopsy of suspicious appearing tissue. (See chapter 12: Endometriosis: Pain or Infertility?)

Endometriosis is found in 20 to 50 percent of infertile women, yet its origins remain an enigma as does its impact on reproduction. Success of surgical treatment to improve fertility is very dependent on the extent of the endometriosis seen at the time of surgery. To be more clear, in women with stage I or II endometriosis, it is estimated that surgery would need to be performed on 12 women for one of them to have a successful pregnancy. This is called the *number needed to treat* (NNT). The NNT is the average number of patients that need to receive a specific treatment for *one* of them to benefit, which in this case is to become pregnant. However, in advanced disease, surgery appears to demonstrate only a modest increase in fertility and only in stage III disease (44 percent pregnancy rate) with less of an effect in stage IV (16.7 percent pregnancy rate). Given these statistics and unless a woman has severe pelvic pain highly suggestive of endometriosis, I do not support performing surgery on an infertile woman just to determine if she has endometriosis. If she has no pelvic pain and her HSG and pelvic ultrasound are normal, a surgery has a very low percentage of finding clinically significant endometriosis. I recommend fertility treatment with IUI or IVF based on her age and male evaluation.

What do we do about ovarian cysts of endometriosis, called endometriomas? During my career, I have seen our society's recommendation swing from advocating for aggressive surgery to conservative treatment. Surely endometriomas represent advanced stage endometriosis. Plus we all believed these cysts would hamper the ovary from responding to fertility medication—so wouldn't it be logical to surgically remove all endometriomas? Yes and no. While it's true, endometriomas reduce ovarian response to fertility injectable medications (gonadotropin stimulation), their removal also reduces ovarian response because the surgery invariably removes healthy ovarian tissue along with the endometrioma. In my opinion, if a woman has already undergone surgery for endometriosis, then additional surgeries for the simple presence of endometriomas is unnecessary, unless she is experiencing significant pain attributed to the disease.

Fibroids

Incredibly, these benign tumors of the uterus, over time, occur in up to 80 percent in African Americans and nearly 70 percent in Caucasians throughout the reproductive years. Fibroids join endometriosis in the association of pain with infertility. Also similar to endometriosis, the optimal management of fibroids regarding your fertility is controversial (see chapter 17: Reproductive Procedures). Apropos, a comprehensive review concluded that the location of fibroids is the overriding factor in deciding whether surgery is necessary to remove them. When fibroids are submucous (i.e., inside the cavity of the uterus where the baby grows), fertility decreases and miscarriage increases, while intramural fibroids (i.e., tumors in the muscle of the uterus) have not been definitively shown to impair fertility. Though an intramural fibroid greater than 4 centimeters (1.6 inches) may impair fertility, current evidence supports surgically removing a fibroid (a procedure called myomectomy) only when it affects the normal shape of your uterine cavity. Outer uterine surface locations of fibroids, called subserosal and pedunculated, should not reduce fertility, though all fibroids may increase obstetric complications.

Polycystic Ovary Syndrome (PCOS)

If I told you there was a hormonal disorder with a major impact on infertility that affects up to 1 in 5 women during their reproductive years, would you know which one? That disorder is PCOS.

Despite being the most prevalent reproductive hormonal disorder, the ideal management of this problem, like the others earlier in this chapter, continues to be debated. In addition to having the reproductive health risks of abnormal uterine bleeding, ovulation dysfunction with subsequent infertility, and uterine cancer, PCOS patients are at a two times higher risk for Metabolic Syndrome, which is a condition that includes abdominal obesity, abnormal lipids, high blood pressure, and prediabetes (for more information, see page 108). Ovulation dysfunction clearly negatively impacts infertility; PCOS is probably the number one cause of infertility. While Metabolic Syndrome can cause serious health risks before and during a pregnancy, only the factor of obesity evidently impairs fertility.

Many studies have suggested that the diabetic medication, metformin, will improve ovulation function in PCOS women, but it's not clear whether metformin improves the chance for a live birth. A natural vitamin-like substance called myo-inositol has been shown to reduce the risk of gestational (in-pregnancy) diabetes. As with many medical therapies, one size does not fit all, and there might be a more selective patient population that may benefit from metformin.

2018 Recommendations from the International Evidence-Based Guideline for the Evaluation and Management of PCOS

- To diagnose PCOS in adults, at least *two* of the following criteria must be met:
  — Ovulation dysfunction with menstrual intervals < 21 or > 35 days or < 8 cycles per year
  — Signs on physical exam or bloodwork of elevated male hormone
  — Polycystic ovaries on ultrasound based on the number of benign tiny cysts and the volume measurement of one or both ovaries

- Although diabetes is not required for the diagnosis, a 2-hour glucose tolerance test is recommended in women who are overweight or obese. BCPs (low dose) are the first-line management for menstrual cycle irregularity and unwanted male-pattern hair growth from elevated male hormone.
- Letrozole, not clomiphene citrate, is the first-line infertility medicine to induce ovulation.
- Gonadotropins, injectable fertility medication, or laparoscopic ovarian diathermy (LOD), a surgery that uses cautery to drill tiny holes into a woman's ovary, is the second-line therapy for ovulation dysfunction.
- IVF is the third-line therapy for ovulation disorders.

For additional information on PCOS, please see chapter 13: Polycystic Ovary Syndrome (PCOS).

In Conclusion

A comprehensive infertility evaluation addresses a woman or couple's risk factors for impaired fertility including prior surgeries, current medications, and lifestyle such as body weight and tobacco use. Pertinent testing can be performed within one month— hysterosalpingogram (HSG) for tubal patency assessment, ovulation testing (either OPK or blood progesterone level), and a sperm analysis. An evidence-based efficient workup can allay anxiety and allow for prompt treatment.

CHAPTER 10

Treatments You Should Avoid

When I go to the auto shop for car repair, I rely completely on the mechanic. After all, what do I know about brakes, engines, batteries, and the like? If the mechanic tells me an item needs repair or replacing because of the risk of the car malfunctioning or of an accident, I simply ask the cost and how long will it take. Does this sound familiar to you?

As patients, we rely on our doctor to perform all appropriate testing to diagnose our problem and to recommend all appropriate treatments to resolve our problem. Infertility patients, in general, are avid online researchers, but consulting "Dr. Google" can induce a sense of comfort, as well as calamity, due to the challenge of finding trustworthy advice.

Caveat Emptor

Only you can be your best champion for fertility care. Your physician and his/her practice should be your best advocate because this is their oath and purpose. Most medical practices are caring, compassionate clinics. The fertility field, unfortunately, has a high risk of patient exploitation due to the high number of cash-paying patients. This is a setup for a medical conflict of interest, that is, the healthcare provider is at risk of recommending certain testing and procedures based on the income they generate to the practice rather than deciding based on medical evidence.

By the end of this chapter, you will know when to avoid ineffective, costly, and possibly harmful treatments that are not supported by medical evidence. By the way, evidence-based medicine is my credo and a recurrent theme throughout this book.

How to Choose Your Fertility Doctor

Consider this advice from the American Board of Obstetrics and Gynecology (ABOG) website: "All certified obstetrician/gynecologists can treat patients with these . . . female disorders to include infertility; . . . however, some physicians have this extra training that qualifies them to take a written and oral test to be certified in these areas."

Board certification in REI means the physician successfully completed rigorous testing for proficiency in the "Care of women who have hormonal or infertility problems," per the ABOG. I fondly remember my three-hour written and three-hour oral examination; actually, it's hard to forget as I continue to intermittently wake up at night screaming out answers! Okay, maybe not, but the exam *was* challenging.

For twenty years, I have committed to following the guidelines of practice by the ASRM while maintaining double board-certification in REI. Why share my credentials—to boast that I am flawless and omniscient in providing infertility care to my patients? Not hardly! Simply stated, anything less than the above qualifications risks substandard, expensive, and risky care along with potentially delayied conception.

Not all physicians who present themselves as fertility specialists have acquired comprehensive training in the field of infertility. As a result, those physicians may (1) order unnecessary hormone testing; (2) misinterpret patients' ovulation function; (3) omit the vital evaluation of the fallopian tubes and sperm; (4) offer fertility medication to ovulating patients without ultrasound monitoring and IUI, which are important components; (5) delay the diagnosis, evaluation, and management of the most common ovulation disorder called PCOS; or (6) perform unnecessary surgical evaluation of your pelvis by a procedure called a laparoscopy. These are some of the more common errors made by healthcare providers with inadequate training in infertility.

Why all the fuss? Because, once you've determined you have a problem conceiving, there are studies to support a shorter time to pregnancy if you immediately establish care with a REI specialist—rather than with a general gynecologist. Based on your age, we recommend natural conception attempts for the following duration prior to an infertility evaluation: (1) women under 35 years of age after one year of TTC; (2) women aged 35 to 39 following six months of attempts; and (3) women 40 years and older after three months. As an infertility patient, you need efficient diagnostic testing and a focused, appropriately aggressive management plan. Most importantly, the physician should validate your frustration and expedite an evaluation, prior to the duration above, if you have infertility risk factors such as a prior pelvic infection, irregular/absent periods, prior chemotherapy, prior infertility, and a known male factor.

A Better Approach: 7 Ways to Avoid Inappropriate Fertility Tests

1. DON'T PERFORM A ROUTINE DIAGNOSTIC LAPAROSCOPY FOR THE EVALUATION OF UNEXPLAINED INFERTILITY.

In the early years of an infertility evaluation, a diagnostic laparoscopy was the rule. This procedure involves placing a telescope through a woman's belly button into her abdomen while she is under anesthesia. As more evidence showed the futility of this procedure without a specific cause, the number of diagnostic laparoscopies for infertility have dramatically declined. What we have learned is when an infertile woman has at least one open fallopian tube and a normal pelvic physical exam and ultrasound, then the likelihood, at the time of surgery, of finding a clinically significant abnormality that will reduce fertility or change a treatment plan is very low.

You also need to be aware that some REI physicians will encourage laparoscopy due to a suspicion of endometriosis, for example because pelvic fluid was seen on a pelvic ultrasound. This is not only unfounded and inappropriate, but it subjects you to an unnecessary and potentially risky surgery.

FYI, endometriosis is a surgical diagnosis, meaning it can only be confirmed by a laparoscopy. If you have no pelvic pain and a normal ultrasound and HSG, there is no medical evidence to compel you to have surgery for the "suspicion" of endometriosis.

2. DON'T PERFORM A POSTCOITAL TEST (PCT) FOR THE EVALUATION OF INFERTILITY.

Truth be told, I have never performed a PCT on an infertility patient nor will I. Why? Because the PCT offers different results from different healthcare providers analyzing the same tests, its predictive value for pregnancy is no better than chance, and pregnancy outcomes are the same whether or not a PCT is included in the infertility evaluation.

The premise of a PCT is to determine the percentage of moving sperm by removing mucus behind the cervix in the vagina after a certain number of hours following intercourse and examining under a microscope. This is where the concern from many of you originated, namely, "Am I killing my partner's sperm with antisperm antibodies?" Short answer—you're not! There is little evidence antisperm antibodies reduce fertility, whether present in the man or woman, so I do not recommend testing.

We used to call a PCT, "the poor man's sperm analysis," meaning one could get an idea of the amount of sperm and the percentage of motility without performing a comprehensive semen exam. By doing a PCT, your fertility specialist may use the results to order more tests and treatments, but this has not increased pregnancy rates. As a result, this is an outdated test that should no longer be offered to evaluate infertility. If your fertility doctor orders a PCT, it is probably time to begin looking for another fertility specialist.

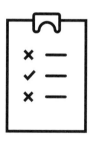

3. DON'T HAVE THROMBOPHILIA OR IMMUNOLOGIC TESTING IF YOU ARE UNDERGOING A ROUTINE INFERTILITY EVALUATION OR SOLELY IF YOU HAVE HAD AN UNSUCCESSFUL IVF CYCLE.

Okay, this is a *huge* area of controversy causing crazy amounts of overtesting and confusion. Thrombophilias are abnormalities of blood coagulation that increase the risk of clotting. They can be congenital (you're born like that) or acquired (you get during your life) proteins in the blood or genetic mutations that predispose patients to clotting. But we're concerned about pregnancy here, so where is the worry and association? Well, the general consensus is that congenital thrombophilias are not associated with infertility or first trimester miscarriage.

What about acquired thrombophilias? Now we're getting somewhere. There are three of these that are significant in the infertility world: lupus anticoagulant, anticardiolipin antibody, and anti-beta 2 glycoprotein. We test for these proteins in the blood only when women have recurrent miscarriage—that's it. There is absolutely no connection between these proteins and the inability to conceive. (More about this testing in the discussion of recurrent miscarriage, in chapter 11: Recurrent Pregnancy Loss).

Since you now understand more about testing for thrombophilias, so let's switch to their cousin, namely, immunologic testing. With decades of research, investigators by now have demonstrated some relationship between immunology factors and infertility. The problem? There just isn't scientific evidence to provide us with guidance on which tests to order, when, and how to treat if there is an immunologic factor found. Although immunological factors may influence early embryo implantation, routine immunology testing for infertility is expensive and does not predict pregnancy.

To make matters worse, unnecessary testing can prompt your doctor to prescribe costly and potentially risky treatment such as injections of a blood thinning heparin-like medication.

Bottom Line: There is no indication to order thrombophilia tests for women with infertility and/or an unsuccessful IVF cycles without recurrent miscarriage or a history of venous thromboembolism (deep vein blood clot). We must also take note that immunologic testing is costly, and there are risks associated with suggested treatments. My advice is to proceed with immunology tests/treatment only if you have consented to be part of a research study because they are not standard of care.

4. ENDOMETRIAL BIOPSY SHOULD NOT BE PERFORMED IN THE ROUTINE EVALUATION OF INFERTILITY.

No office diagnostic procedure breaks my heart more than when I perform an endometrial biopsy. Why? Because it hurts most women to the point of tears. Believe me, I have tried everything I know: before the procedure injecting liquid numbing medicine (lidocaine), having her take anti-inflammatory medications, and even prescribing sedatives. These methods do provide some relief and patients vary in their pain tolerance. Fortunately the biopsy is brief and then we allow the patient to remain reclined with the addition of a heating pad to her lower tummy as needed.

What are the reasons for performing an endometrial biopsy? In the infertility world, there are a few valid indications: evaluating women with PCOS to determine if their uterine lining has precancerous or cancerous cells due to chronic abnormal uterine bleeding; looking for chronic inflammation; or important embryo implantation proteins. Endometrial receptive tests can report the most optimal timing to transfer an embryo into your uterus and can also check if the lining has chronic inflammation, called endometritis, which has been seen in recurrent miscarriage patients.

When should you not have the test? For any other reason given to you besides the ones above, with the rare exception of determining development of the lining in preparation for a frozen embryo replacement (more on this in chapter 17: Reproductive Procedures). Otherwise an endometrial biopsy should not be part of an infertility evaluation.

How did the endometrial biopsy become erroneously part of an infertility evaluation? First a little background. During a woman's natural cycle, the lining of the uterus (endometrium) thickens from ovarian estradiol (estrogen). Following ovulation of the egg from the ovary's follicle cyst, progesterone is produced from the newly termed corpus luteum cyst (see sidebar Why Do You Get a Period? on page 84). Progesterone's effect on the endometrium is exquisitely synchronized for embryo implantation. The embryo needs to make it to the uterine cavity by 5 to 6 days after fertilization for a successful pregnancy.

In 1950, in a classic medical article called "Dating the Endometrial Biopsy" published in *Obstetrical & Gynecological Survey*, Drs. Noyes, Hertig, and Rock microscopically studied the luteal phase of the endometrium. The luteal phase (the two weeks following ovulation until menses) was described to determine the actual appearance of endometrial tissue coinciding with the specific day after ovulation (i.e., day 4, day 6, etc.) This is called endometrial dating. My specialty, in the earlier days, felt dating was vital to fertility. Alas, it's another theory that eventually was refuted. You see, at times, both fertile and infertile women have since been shown to have abnormal dating.

The luteal phase is dominated by the hormone progesterone, and its level begins to rise at ovulation, peaks one week later, and then falls if no pregnancy occurs. As a result, due to its fluctuations, a random blood progesterone level is of no value to judge a good luteal phase. Any blood level above 3 ng/mL (3 nanograms per milliliter) is all that is needed to presume ovulation; a higher number is meaningless and not a measure of a good ovulation.

WHY DO YOU GET A PERIOD?

A woman gets a period because she's not pregnant. You read that right and it's not a "duh" statement. Every month, if you have regular menstrual intervals and ovulate, your body, specifically your uterus, prepares for a pregnancy. The brain's pituitary gland at ovulation sends an LH signal to stimulate the ovarian follicle cyst to ovulate (release an egg). LH continues to stimulate the ovarian cyst, now called a corpus luteum, to make progesterone. Progesterone, the hormone of pregnancy (think "pro-gestation), changes your endometrium into a "welcome mat" for the embryo. But, here's a catch: LH stimulation will last for only eight to ten days; otherwise, the corpus luteum resorbs (breaks down and assimilates) and progesterone levels plummet.

What rescues the corpus luteum? Well, it's every fertility patient's dream hormone—beta hCG or human chorionic gonadotropin: The beta part of hCG distinguishes it from the pituitary hormones that share the same alpha part, namely TSH, FSH, and LH; and "dream" because detection of this hormone in the urine or blood means pregnancy!

When the corpus luteum resorbs and progesterone levels drop, it means two things: You are not pregnant and your period is near. The endometrium responds to a withdrawal of progesterone by causing contractions that cut off the blood supply of the superficial layer of the linings resulting in shedding and your period.

To get back to "you get a period because you're not pregnant"—it's somewhat like the chicken and the egg. You cannot maintain your uterine lining without progesterone and you cannot maintain your progesterone unless you are pregnant. So you get your period because progesterone levels drop since you are not pregnant.

5. ROUTINE SERUM PROLACTIN TESTING IN A WOMAN WITH REGULAR MENSES, OVULATION, AND LACK OF NIPPLE DISCHARGE IS ALSO OF NO VALUE.

A bit of background: Many fertility clinics offer onsite (called "in-house") hormone testing to provide important same-day results to their patients who are undergoing treatment cycles and may need medication adjustment. These labs offer convenience of rapid results and, appropriately, another revenue stream for the practice.

The problem lies in the potential conflict of interest—performing hormone testing that generates revenue for the practice but is without medical evidence to support its need as part of the initial general infertility evaluation. Examples of these hormones are prolactin and DHEAS (a weak male hormone). Unfortunately, I have seen patients who have the FSH blood test (for ovarian age) repeated almost monthly. This is not only unnecessary and costly, but FSH has been replaced by a newer ovarian age blood test called AMH.

Prolactin is a brain pituitary hormone that really serves an unknown purpose outside of pregnancy. When you are not pregnant, elevations of prolactin can cause menstrual cycle irregularity, ovulation dysfunction, recurrent miscarriage, and milky nipple discharge (galactorrhea). During pregnancy, prolactin aids in preparing the breast for lactation (breast feeding).

Many fertility practices obtain a prolactin levels as part of the routine infertility evaluation. However, unless you have galactorrhea, irregular menstrual cycles, or recurrent miscarriage, you gain no benefit to having this blood test.

6. HSG SHOULD BE PERFORMED ONCE AT THE BEGINNING OF THE INFERTILITY EVALUATION AND REPEATED ONLY WITH RARE EXCEPTION.

HSG is the acronym for hysterosalpingography—"hystero" means uterus; "salpingo" means tube; and graphy means description. This outpatient test is performed in a radiology center or your fertility doctor's office and is without anesthesia. To briefly describe an HSG, contrast dye is injected into a woman's uterus through her cervix. An X-ray machine, called a C-arm, takes photos by fluoroscopy, which is a continuous X-ray like a movie to see motion of the dye. The contrast dye appears clear outside the body, but this liquid allows a great contrast to outline the uterus and tubes. An HSG can result in varying degrees of mild to severe discomfort. By taking anti-inflammatory medication prior to the procedure and having the physician inject the dye slowly, your procedure should be much more tolerable.

WHAT DOES THIS TEST TELL YOU?

The basic information gained from the HSG is whether the inside of the uterus (uterine cavity) is normal and if both fallopian tubes are open. A normal uterine cavity has no area where the dye is interrupted with "filling defects." If the uterine cavity has defects, this is usually due to an abnormality within the cavity that prevents the dye from evenly distributing; examples of such abnormalities are endometrial polyps, uterine fibroids, and intrauterine adhesions. The tubes also should demonstrate a steady flow of dye throughout their length and spread evenly in the pelvis to signify they are open. Abnormalities in the tubes are typically a blockage: at the beginning, closest to the uterus (called proximal occlusion; in the mid-portion of the tube, often seen after a woman has had her tubes tied and unsuccessfully reversed; or at the end, particularly dilated, called a hydrosalpinx (see chapter 10).

REASONS TO REPEAT AN HSG:
- Reproductive surgery involving the uterus and/or fallopian tubes
- Ectopic pregnancy
- Up to one year of infertility with a new partner
- A pelvic and/or STI
- Advanced endometriosis

Earlier in this chapter, I talked about caveat emptor due to the potential conflict of interest when a physician's recommendation for a test or procedure is influenced by the revenue generated. Well, an HSG is another one of those potential issues, especially when the medical practice owns the C-arm. If your doctor recommends a repeat HSG after the one done at your initial evaluation, then check the above list before jumping into another fun-filled procedure.

OIL VS. WATER-BASED DYE FOR HSG

During most of the 20th century, the HSG procedure included the use of oil-based dye (OBD) to light up the uterus and fallopian tubes. Toward the latter part of that century and throughout the 21st, water contrast dye (WCD) has replaced OBD. Why? Mainly due to concerns of oil slowly being absorbed in the body and able to remain for months to years as well as a life-threatening rare complication of emboli (travel in the bloodstream to potentially clog a major blood vessel). Controversy lingered over whether OBD had a therapeutic effect on improving pregnancy rates following HSG. More recently, interest has been renewed in OBD as a study reported in the *New England Journal of Medicine* in 2017 showed a 10 percent increase in pregnancy rates using OBD over WCD, meaning 10 women would need to have the HSG for one more woman to get pregnant. In my opinion, the use of OBD appears to have a small but therapeutic effect on fertility, although most centers do not offer this option.

YOU WERE RIGHT!

All this writing about HSGs brings me to remember a patient, let's call her Kathleen, who was extremely anxious about having the procedure. To be clear, most patients show up with various degrees of anxiety and caution over having the HSG. But Kathleen was nearly hyperventilating. All my assurances, explanations, and jokes were failing. So, I finally offered this, "I am guaranteeing you that you will not have anywhere near the degree of discomfort you are anticipating and dreading." This finally got to her and, though skeptical, she agreed to proceed. You see, medicine is just never a guarantee. Try as we might, we can never predict an outcome.

Like the endometrial biopsy, an HSG can be very uncomfortable and even downright painful. The key, in my experience, is to numb the cervix before placing a clamp-like instrument on it; inject the dye slowly; and talk to the patient during the entire procedure describing what is happening and have her view the monitor to see her uterus and tubes.

More about the importance of injecting slowly—the uterus is composed of smooth muscle as opposed to skeletal muscle that can voluntary be moved and controlled. A smooth muscle responds to expansion by contracting. Think of the heart—blood fills it, the chamber expands, and then it contracts to send the blood onward. The same goes for the uterus. If the dye is pushed into the cavity quickly, the uterus will expand and contract resulting in an intense cramp felt by the woman.

So how did Kathleen do? Well I followed all the tips above and injected especially very slow. Without exaggeration, I really felt my reputation was at stake. Fortunately, the procedure ended with her exclamation, "that wasn't bad!" She even went one step further to thank me by mailing me a card with the title, "you were right." I can't imagine any greater joy then performing a procedure on an anxious patient whose high expectations of pain never materialized.

7. USING OVARIAN AGE TESTING TO DETERMINE THE NEED FOR IVF OR EGG DONATION.

The absolute best predictor of the chance for pregnancy for a woman, as I tell all my patients, is your age. Dreaded by some and despised by all, your age is the single most defining factor in giving you a realistic percentage regarding your likelihood for pregnancy. No test reveals your ovarian age marker, score, blood level, index or any calculation, chart, graph, spreadsheet, or anything else that beats how old you are. I know there are labs trying to "sell" you and doctors on the best ovarian age tests. But, like it or not, nothing gets better reproductively with age, and for that matter, nothing does except maybe wine.

This is not omitting the male contribution. More information is being reported that reveals the negative reproductive effects with advancing paternal age including infertility, miscarriage, preterm birth, birth defects, autism, and schizophrenia, particularly for fathers above ages 40 to 45.

Ovarian age testing should optimally be used by your physician only to gauge your dose of infertility medication (the more aging, the higher the dose to stimulate the ovary) and to estimate the number of eggs retrieved during your IVF cycle (the more aging, the less the number). As I discussed earlier in chapter 2 with my **SWAT** analysis, random ovarian age testing does not predict your live birth rate (i.e., your chance to deliver a baby).

> Your physician should not be routinely obtaining blood levels of FSH, LH, and estradiol for two reasons: For ovarian age testing, FSH levels are unreliable as they fluctuate monthly, and LH and estradiol levels have limited to no value in this circumstance. AMH, along with the ultrasound AFC, is a more reliable and earlier predictor of ovarian age and has replaced FSH for more than ten years.

In Conclusion

In whatever area of medicine you are a patient, you must be proactive and vigilant during your care to find a physician/clinic who is your advocate. I see so many patients who visit my office wanting a second opinion because they were concerned the recommendation from their fertility doctors "just didn't feel right"—such as

- You have endometriosis and need IVF.
- Your sperm analysis is abnormal, so you need IVF.
- Your AMH is low so you need egg donation.

In my career, I have never told a patient that they need IVF. Why? Because IVF is no guarantee and there are always family building options, such as IUI, surrogacy, adoption, and even IVF with egg donation.

If you are unclear or uncomfortable regarding a proposed test or treatment plan, you should always ask your healthcare providers questions or seek a second opinion.

CHAPTER 11

Recurrent Pregnancy Loss (RPL)

66 "I am sorry, you lost your baby." No other words could come close to the trauma these seven simple words cause for me when I say them—or for a patient to hear them. I pray you will never experience this anguish. Yet, statistically, if you are a woman less than age 30, your chance of a first trimester loss is 10 percent; over age 40, it's about 33 percent or up to 1 in 3 women. You, a family member, or friend, have possibly faced this agony.

RPL is a devastating problem affecting up to 5 percent of the population. Of all the patients I see for infertility, those with RPL are the most emotionally tortured. While most women are rejoicing their positive pregnancy test, a patient with RPL is on guard with worry for every minute of the first three months of her pregnancy and possibly longer.

RPL is defined as two or more clinical pregnancies lost at less than 20 weeks gestation. Two losses occur in 5 percent of women, while three or more losses occurs in 1 to 2 percent of you. Clinical pregnancies are distinct from preclinical (or biochemical) pregnancies: A clinical pregnancy is at a stage where it is visible inside the uterine cavity by ultrasound; a chemical pregnancy is at such an early stage that it cannot be viewed by ultrasound and only confirmed by a blood or urine test for the pregnancy hormone hCG. A clinical pregnancy loss also differs from a pregnancy loss due to an ectopic pregnancy, which is an abnormal pregnancy implanted outside the normal uterine location, or a pregnancy of unknown location (PUL), which is an abnormal pregnancy whose implantation location cannot be confirmed.

When to Evaluate

If you have experienced this tragic loss, you probably have been told the most common reason is a chromosomal abnormality of the embryo, which occurs in up to 75 percent of cases. However, the more pregnancy losses you have, the more likely each miscarried embryo was chromosomally normal.

Studies have shown the results of a comprehensive evaluation for RPL is the same when testing begins following two or following three or more losses. As a result, many clinicians and most of you prefer testing after two losses, particularly in women above age 34, as well as those with significant risk factors. Increasing evidence shows men over age 40 also have a higher rate of contributing to miscarriages.

RPL Cause, Percentage, and Evaluation

The accepted causes of RPL are genetic, anatomic, hormonal, and acquired thrombophilias. Each of these causes will be described in more detail below. The evaluation is not complicated and should be limited to testing that is supported by solid medical evidence. Unfortunately, as an RPL patient, you are desperate for an answer and for treatment. This places you at risk of exploitation with excessive testing and unsubstantiated therapy. The following are the causes of RPL and their percentages of likelihood.

1. GENETIC (LESS THAN 5 PERCENT)

Blood tests for chromosomal analysis for you and the biological father are essential because we are looking for an inherited genetic contribution called a translocation. (Normally, all the cells of a healthy person have 23 pairs of chromosomes: 22 non-sex plus XX or XY determining female or male gender, respectively.)

Translocations represent a rearrangement of a piece of genetic material from one numbered chromosome to another, but the total, normal amount of DNA is present. During fertilization, the sperm and egg (each with 23 individual chromosomes) interact and combine to return to 23 pairs of chromosomes. When either the sperm or egg contain a translocation, several different inheritance patterns for the embryo result:

— Normal
— Balanced translocation
— Unbalanced translocation

Simply having a translocation does not ensure a miscarriage unless the embryo is unbalanced; rarely, such a baby is carried to term.

The overall cumulative live birth rate for couples with a balanced translocation is roughly 55 to 75 percent, with no improvement from the addition of IVF with chromosome testing of the embryos prior to embryo transfer into your uterus. This is called IVF with PGT-A. PGT-A is preimplantation genetic testing for aneuploidy, an abnormality in the number of chromosomes. While PGT remains controversial, embryo chromosome testing with subsequent transfer may reduce the risk of miscarriage.

I should add that while translocations are a rare cause of RPL, you are more likely to be diagnosed with this condition when you have intermittent live births between the miscarriages rather than continuous miscarriages without ever having a child.

2. ANATOMIC (15 PERCENT)

Abnormalities of the uterine cavity have been shown to reduce the ability for the embryo to implant and to increase the risk of miscarriage. Problems you will encounter will either be congenital or acquired.

CONGENITAL	ACQUIRED
Septate uterus—residual tissue in the midline of the cavity from abnormal development as an embryo	Endometrial polyps—benign overgrowths of the normal lining, easily removed
	Fibroids (benign tumors) that affect the uterine cavity;
	Asherman's syndrome—intrauterine scarring

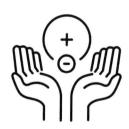

To identify these uterine abnormalities, we can view your uterine cavity in three ways:

- **Hysteroscopy** involves passing a thin telescope inside the uterus while saline is gently injected into your uterus; this is the gold standard evaluation tool given its direct visualization of the uterus. This procedure can be performed in the office or hospital based on patient preference and complexity of the surgery.
- **HSG** injects contrast dye into your uterine cavity under fluoroscopic X-rays, showing the inside of the uterus for any potential defects and whether your fallopian tubes are open.
- **Saline infusion sonogram (SIS)** images your uterine cavity by injecting saline under ultrasound into your uterus to look for polyps, fibroids, scarring, or a congenital septum, all of which can and should be surgically corrected.

A uterine septum can be mild or severe, based on its depth. The Müllerian system forms the uterus and fallopian tubes very early in the embryo. Some Müllerian anomalies have no impact on miscarriage but do increase your risk of a breach presentation of the baby and preterm labor/delivery. A uterine septum increases the risk of miscarriage, and the surgery to restore the uterine cavity to normal is called a metroplasty (incising [cutting] the septum). A review of a large number of studies concluded that congenital uterine anomalies were present in 4.3 percent (range from 2.7 percent to 16.7 percent) of the general population of fertile women and in 12.6 percent (range from 1.8 percent to 37.6 percent) of you with RPL (two or more consecutive losses).

Having a uterine septum is associated with a high incidence of pregnancy loss (44.3 percent loss). Fortunately, correction of the septum may have beneficial effects (live birth rate 83.2 percent, range from 77.4 percent to 90.9 percent).

Special mention should be made about your having fibroids and their impact on miscarriage. First, these benign uterine tumors are very common in women, with an overall incidence of 40 percent to 60 percent by age 35 and 70 percent to 80 percent by age 50. Surgery to remove fibroids (myomectomy) is recommended if the fibroid is distorting or changing the normal shape of the uterine cavity. To be clear, however, there is no definitive evidence that you should have your fibroid(s) removed to reduce miscarriage and improve fertility if your uterine cavity is normal.

One special consideration for myomectomy, even when you have a normal uterine cavity, is when the fibroids they prevent us from being able to retrieve your eggs for egg freezing or IVF.

About 22 to 32 percent of you who have fibroids will experience growth of your fibroids during pregnancy, almost exclusively in the first trimester. In 10 to 30 percent of your pregnancies, complications that can occur due to fibroids (see table Complications During Pregnancies Due to Fibroids, below) include miscarriage, preterm labor, and preterm premature rupture of membranes.

COMPLICATIONS DURING PREGNANCIES DUE TO FIBROIDS	
Miscarriage	Placental abruption
Preterm labor	Postpartum hemorrhage
Preterm premature rupture of membranes	Abnormal presentation of baby, e.g. breach

Another anatomic abnormality is chronic endometritis (CE). CE has been associated in 27 percent of you with recurrent miscarriage (and in 14 percent of patients with recurrent implantation failure following IVF with embryo transfer).

Occurring in 10 percent of all women, CE is not an active infection but has been associated with recurrent miscarriage and may play a role in implantation failure. Typically, you are unaware you even have CE as it poses no consequences to your health. Symptoms, if present, are vague and consist of abnormal uterine bleeding and pelvic pain. We diagnose this condition by office endometrial biopsy. If you are found to have CE, we prescribe doxycycline for 14 days and recommend a repeat biopsy to demonstrate resolution of CE. If CE remains present or recurs, we can change your prescription to amoxicillin/clavulanate and then repeat the endometrial biopsy.

3. THROMBOPHILIAS (15 PERCENT)

This is the area that causes the most confusion for you and even physicians: antiphospholipid antibodies (APA). These APAs are proteins in the blood that can cause clotting and miscarriage. Medical studies only support obtaining these three blood tests: lupus anticoagulant (a misnomer and not diagnostic test for Lupus), anticardiolipin antibody, and anti-beta 2 glycoprotein. All of these are looking for the antiphospholipid syndrome (APS) as recommended by a 2006 International Consensus Statement.

APS's consequences include RPL, thrombosis (blood clots), and/or autoimmune low platelets. APA are only of clinical significance when lupus anticoagulant, anticardiolipin antibodies, or anti-beta2 glycoprotein remain elevated three months apart following two separate laboratory blood tests. Once a laboratory and clinical criteria are met, APS is diagnosed.

If you have been diagnosed with APS, unfortunately, there is an up to a 90 percent fetal loss rate without intervention. Treatment includes a low-dose aspirin (81 mg daily) and low dose heparin (5,000 to 10,000 units subcutaneously every 12 hours) or low molecular weight heparin daily throughout the first trimester of pregnancy. These medications are thought to help prevent blood clotting (thrombosis) in the placenta. The treatment of APS, although not completely understood, has been shown to improve the outcome of your pregnancy; however, fetal losses continue in some women despite adequate therapy.

Another autoimmune issue in which you should be aware is thyroid peroxidase antibodies (TPO). These are thyroid antibodies circulating in your blood that may increase your risk of miscarriage and reduce live birth rates. If your TSH (thyroid-stimulating hormone) is in the normal range and you have a positive TPO, recent evidence suggests low dose thyroid hormone may improve fertility and reduce this risk of miscarriage.

4. HORMONAL (20 PERCENT)

In this category, we evaluate you for

— Thyroid dysfunction with a blood TSH level

We regulate an unstable thyroid with thyroxine (natural thyroid hormone) for more strict control of your TSH level during pregnancy for the optimal level of less than 2.5 mU/L, apparently improving cognitive development of your baby, although this is under enormous debate in the medical literature.

If you have thyroid disfunction your TSH should be checked, at the least, in each trimester of pregnancy and adjusted accordingly.

— Prolactin elevations.

Before initiating medication to restore your prolactin to normal, we often will check your pituitary with an MRI (magnetic resonance imaging) to ensure there is no large growth that would compel us to check other hormones.

We normalize your elevated prolactin level by prescribing a medication that works to increase your body's dopamine, called cabergoline, and should be discontinued in pregnancy.

— Hemoglobin A1c to screen for diabetes.

Uncontrolled diabetes cannot only risk miscarriage but it also increases complications of diabetes in your pregnancy along with birth defects of your baby.

Also, while a shortened second half of your menstrual cycle (luteal phase) is associated with miscarriage, there is no benefit to evaluate for a so-called "luteal phase defect." You may read about this online, but medical studies do not agree how to test for this condition or that it is a real condition.

5. UNEXPLAINED (50 PERCENT)

The fifth but most common reason for RPL is unexplained. This is the good news/bad news cause: Good because it means a natural successful birth still may occur—up to 70 to 80 percent of you may have a baby over the 10 years from first seeing a specialist; Bad because there is no definitive abnormality to treat.

Surprisingly, close monitoring of you and your pregnancy by a medical staff with supportive and empathic care throughout the first trimester (the so-called "TLC effect") has been demonstrated in medical studies to improve your pregnancy outcome. For all of you with RPL, we prescribe natural progesterone vaginal suppositories liberally; this supplementation has been shown to help you if you have experienced four or more losses. Progesterone support in the form of injections of 17 hydroxyprogesterone caproate weekly during the first trimester has been shown to reduce loss if you have bleeding in the first trimester.

The advanced technology of IVF with PGT-A for embryo biopsy and analysis of the chromosomes of the embryo may reduce miscarriage. Although there is much enthusiasm for PGT, overall pregnancy rates over time appear to be similar whether a couple tries naturally vs. IVF with PGT-A, but the latter may shorten time to pregnancy with a reduced risk of miscarriage.

Seven Surprising Facts about Recurrent Pregnancy Loss (RPL)

1. FOLIC ACID DECREASES EMBRYO CHROMOSOMAL ABNORMALITIES AND MISCARRIAGE.

Folic acid in doses of at least 0.4 mg daily have long been advocated to reduce spina bifida and neural tube defects in newborns. It is optimal for you to begin folic acid for several months prior to conception attempts. There is also now evidence folic acid may help treat RPL by reducing the chance for chromosomal abnormalities of the embryo. I recommend 0.8 to 1 mg daily.

2. EARLY PROGESTERONE SUPPORT MAY REDUCE BIOCHEMICAL MISCARRIAGE.

A biochemical pregnancy loss is defined as a miscarriage prior to detection/confirmation by pelvic ultrasound. This type of pregnancy and miscarriage occurs more commonly than realized since many of you may experience a late period without ever checking a pregnancy test. Natural progesterone (unlike synthetic) has long been used to treat and/or prevent miscarriage. Though there is no evidence for its value when initiated in pregnancies after five weeks, you may receive a benefit when given earlier in pregnancy.

3. THERE IS NO BENEFIT TO USING ASPIRIN AND/OR HEPARIN TO TREAT UNEXPLAINED RECURRENT MISCARRIAGES (RM).

Despite many proponents of this approach, especially on the internet, the use of aspirin and/or heparin has convincingly been shown to *not* improve live birth rates when the cause of RPL is unknown. Other attempted therapies such as white blood cell transfusion and intralipid infusion should also not be prescribed and offered only as part of experimental research protocols after full informed consent is provided to you regarding the risks.

4. INHERITED THROMBOPHILIAS ARE NOT ASSOCIATED WITH RPL AND SHOULD NOT BE TESTED.

Screening for Factor V (Leiden mutation), Factor II (Prothrombin G20210A), and MTHFR (Methylenetetrahydrofolate reductase) have not been shown to increase RPL although many physicians and patients request testing for them. No treatment (such as aspirin and/or heparin) improves the live birth rate. Only *acquired* thrombophilias (lupus anticoagulant, anticardiolipin antibody, and anti-beta 2 glycoprotein) benefit from treatment resulting in improved live birth rates.

5. CLOSE MONITORING AND EMPATHIC CARE IMPROVE OUTCOME.

For unknown reasons, clinics providing close monitoring, emotional support, and education to moms with unexplained RPL report higher live birth rates compared with women not receiving this level of care. We have known this phenomenon for many years. I have seen firsthand the success of this approach but cannot begin to explain it, except for a benefit in the dramatic reduction in mom's stress every time she sees the ultrasound showing the embryo's heart beating.

The close monitoring protocol we use is early pregnancy testing by blood hCG level and then repeating twice weekly until ultrasound monitoring begins at an EGA of 6 weeks. Once a viable intrauterine pregnancy (IUP) is confirmed, we ask you to return every 10 days for repeat ultrasounds until 10 weeks when you are returned to your obstetrician. We also are available 24/7 for phone calls of your concern. For example, if you have some vaginal bleeding/spotting or abdominal pain, even if you dreamt it, we bring you in to the office right away for an exam and ultrasound for reassurance.

I don't want to misrepresent this close monitoring protocol and its association with stress.

This is clearly not saying your RPL is all due to stress or even mostly due to stress or even somewhat due to stress. That is unequivocally unfair to you if people share their unsubstantiated advice to "just relax." Fortunately, medical evidence has supported this TLC effect and we have had reasonable success!

6. BEHAVIOR CHANGES REDUCE MISCARRIAGE.

Believe it or not, certain lifestyle choices you make cannot only affect your ability to conceive but also to maintain carrying the pregnancy. The major ones to address:
- Weight, calculated by BMI
- Tobacco use
- Caffeine intake

Elevations in BMI and cigarette smoking both increase the risk of miscarriage. As a result, a healthy BMI and eliminating tobacco use reduce the risk of pregnancy loss. Caffeine may also be a culprit. Drinking excessive amounts of caffeine (more than two equivalent cups of coffee or 200 mg caffeine from any source per day) also increases miscarriage. However, recent evidence has raised doubts on the negative effects of caffeine.

7. FERTILITY MEDICATIONS, IUI, AND STANDARD IVF DO NOT IMPROVE OUTCOME.

When you are diagnosed with unexplained RPL, you often feel compelled to undergo fertility treatment. Unfortunately, medications, IUI, and even IVF have not been shown to improve the chance for live birth if you have RPL. However, the advanced technology of IVF with chromosomal testing of embryos prior to transfer (PGT-A) allows for the identification of normal embryos. This process has been shown to lower the miscarriage rate to less than 10%.

In Conclusion

In cases of RPL, I recommend obtaining chromosomal testing of the woman and her male partner, viewing the uterine cavity and performing an endometrial biopsy, and blood testing for thyroid, prolactin, blood sugar control, and acquired thrombophilias.

The good news is, when the cause is unexplained, you have a 70 to 80 percent chance of a spontaneous live birth within the next ten years from diagnosis. The impact of a lost pregnancy can be one of the hardest events to endure. By further understanding, knowing how to diagnose, and treating proven causes of RPL, we can hopefully prevent this heartbreaking and devastating problem.

CHAPTER 12

Endometriosis: Pain or Infertility?

The term "chronic" can be defined as long-lasting and difficult to rid. This meaning can represent both endometriosis and infertility. These two conditions are related in that they both can cause chronic disruptions in your life: endometriosis through physical pain; infertility through emotional pain.

Yet, these two diseases are much more closely associated, that is, endometriosis is associated with and accepted as a cause of infertility; and infertility, through its incessant (or continuous) monthly menstruation without stopping for a pregnancy, may increase the risk of endometriosis. Why? From the most prevailing theory of "retrograde menstruation." This premise originates from the age-old presumption that monthly menstrual cycles allows for the continuous flow of blood not only out of the vagina but also back through the tubes to potentially implant on the ovaries and throughout the pelvis. A disease affecting at least 6 to 10 percent of all women reading this book, endometriosis is found in 25 to 50 percent of women with infertility, while 30 to 50 percent of women with endometriosis have infertility. When your fallopian tubes are open and if your pelvic anatomy is normal, endometriosis and infertility have an unclear relationship of cause and effect.

Endometriosis has always been presumed to develop by the famous *Sampson's theory of retrograde menstruation*, stemming from the backwards flow of menstrual blood. This theory suggests that the shed uterine lining, consisting of endometrial cells, attaches to the lining of the abdominal cavity (also called the peritoneum) and creates inflammation, which is then followed by implantation and the growth of the endometrial cells—the most common victim is the ovary. What's more, like all uterine lining tissue, endometriosis is estrogen sensitive, meaning that any medications or condition that increases estrogen can worsen the disease.

Sampson's theory certainly makes sense, but we know that all women have some degree of retrograde menstruation back through the tubes into the pelvic cavity. So, why don't all of you get this disease? We just don't know. But when you have advanced endometriosis, you can have extensive scar tissue formation, blocked fallopian tubes, and blood-filled ("chocolate") ovarian cysts called endometriomas. This disease seems to be more common in those of you with congenital variations in the shape of your uterus, called *Müllerian anomalies*, which can result in menstrual flow blockage that increases retrograde flow and thereby the cycle described above.

Other risk factors you may have that more likely results in endometriosis:

- A young age at menarche (first menses)
- Shorter menstrual intervals
- Smoking tobacco
- Drinking alcohol
- A low BMI

In the United States, up to $56 billion is annually spent on endometriosis-related health care costs and loss of employment days. Classic symptoms (aside from infertility) include

- Chronic pelvic pain: 71 to 87 percent of these women have endometriosis
- Dysmenorrhea (painful periods)
- Dyspareunia (painful intercourse)
- Dysuria (painful urination) and dyschezia (painful bowel movement), if present, usually occur during menstruation

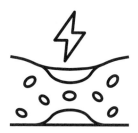

Options if Fertility Is Not Desired

If having a baby is not your immediate goal, treatment options for endometriosis include (in order of relatively least to most effective):

- BCPs (The combined hormones of synthetic estrogen and progesterone have been long used to manage the pain of endometriosis, but the exact method and true effectiveness is not clear.)
- Progestins (Synthetic progesterone medications suppress estrogen and help relieve the painful symptoms of endometriosis.)
- Male hormone (androgenic) drugs, such as danocrine (This drug has been effective at treating women with endometriosis since the 1970s. However, its many androgenic [male-like] side effects, including weight gain, increased body hair, acne, plus potentially irreversible deepening of the voice, has made the use of danocrine fall out of favor.)
- Gonadotropin-releasing hormone agonist (GnRH agonist), such as luprolide (This injectable medication has been effective in relieving the symptoms of endometriosis in women for over 20 years. Due to estrogen suppression, the drug places women in a "medical-menopause" condition, resulting in unwanted side effects including hot flashes, vaginal dryness, and bone loss, which limits the medications duration of use.)
- Gonadotropin-releasing hormone antagonist (GnRH antagonist), such as elagolix (Like luprolide, this new drug results in a rapid suppression of endometriosis but comes in a pill form. It shows great promise in treating painful symptoms of endometriosis.)
- Surgery, usually minimally invasive advanced laparoscopy, to remove all visible endometriosis and scar tissue that may be contributing to pain. (Unfortunately, not all endometriosis can be removed as 20 percent of normal appearing tissue seen at laparoscopic surgery may still have endometriosis as determined under the microscope after the tissue is biopsied.)

Endometriosis-related Infertility

If you're TTC and have been told you have, or may have, endometriosis, then this section is for you.

You should first know that endometriosis can only be truly diagnosed at the time of surgery. Only ultrasound or MRI of a classic appearing ovarian cyst of endometriosis (endometrioma) can help you with a diagnosis preoperatively. Endometriosis is staged by how much spread there is in the pelvis and how deep the invasion into tissue: I-minimal, II-mild, III-moderate, IV-severe. The more advanced the stage, the more anatomic distortion of reproductive anatomy and, presumably, infertility.

Stage III and stage IV endometriosis do have a reduced fertility rate, which may be improved following surgery. In stage III/IV, surgery appears more beneficial. Cumulative pregnancy rates for infertile patients followed for up to two years after laparoscopy or laparotomy (open surgery) are 45 percent and 63 percent, respectively. Advanced endometriosis may reduce the pregnancy rate with IVF.

BETWEEN A ROCK AND A HARD PLACE

Ovarian cysts of endometriosis (endometriomas) can reduce the ovarian follicle development as a response to stimulating fertility medications; however, surgically removing these cysts (cystectomies) results in the problem of reduced follicle response. Why? Because cystectomies will also remove some healthy ovarian tissue. Consideration of ovarian cystectomy would be for a painful or undiagnosed complex ovarian cyst that is seen on pelvic ultrasound. Unless you are having significant symptoms from a diagnosed endometriomas, then I would not recommend surgery but simply monitor intermittently while TTC.

One caveat: Having an endometrioma, you are a slightly higher risk of developing a pelvic infection following an egg retrieval. I recommend an antibiotic immediately prior to the procedure.

Currently, in low stages of endometriosis, there is poor evidence for surgical benefit to improve your fertility. The NNT when undergoing laparoscopic resection of mild endometriosis for the result of getting pregnant would be a total of 12 women to have the procedure for one to have the positive outcome of a successful pregnancy.

As a result, if you have a normal pelvic examination, no pelvic pain (including painful menses or intercourse), and normal pelvic ultrasound and HSG (for tubal patency), I am against attempts at a surgical evaluation with laparoscopy to diagnose suspected endometriosis because it is not supported by medical evidence.

Treatment of endometriosis-related infertility, as a woman, should be based on your age. Younger than age 35, you could begin with fertility medication with IUI for three to no more than six cycles is reasonable. Older than age 35, particularly following prior fertility treatment and years of infertility, you should consider either three cycles of medication with IUI or going direct to IVF. While IVF pregnancy rates appear lower in women with endometriosis, surgery prior to IVF does not improve your outcome and is unnecessary for fertility.

ENDOMETRIOSIS FERTILITY INDEX (EFI)

If you want to know your chance of pregnancy based on surgical findings and treatment of endometriosis, then EFI might very well be your best friend. In 2010, the EFI score was published to help you estimate your chance of a non-IVF pregnancy following endometriosis surgery. On the worksheet, you enter your patient history, which is your age, years infertile, and prior pregnancies, and your doctor enters the subsequent surgical scores, which are the least functional result of your endometriosis surgery based on fallopian tube function, amount of damage caused, and how widespread the disease is. The history score total and the surgery score total are added together and the result is compared to a graph that estimates your chance of a non-IVF pregnancy over 36 months. This may help you decide how aggressive you would like to be with fertility medications based on your prognosis for pregnancy.

In Conclusion

If you are symptomatic from advanced stage endometriosis and TTC, surgery is a reasonable option for potentially improving your pregnancy chance as well as hopefully experiencing much needed pain relief. The impact of low-stage endometriosis on fertility is not definitively proven, so I recommend you avoid surgery unless you have significant pelvic symptoms, an abnormal pelvic ultrasound, or one or both blocked fallopian tubes.

CHAPTER 13

Polycystic Ovary Syndrome (PCOS)

M uch, more prevalent than you might imagine, the impact of PCOS on women's health is profound and the numbers are staggering:

- PCOS affects up to 20 percent of women.
- 70 to 80 percent of infertility patients are diagnosed with PCOS.
- 80 percent of ovulation disorders are due to PCOS.
- At least one-third of you wait longer than 2 years and almost half need to see three or more health professionals before you are diagnosed with PCOS.
- PCOS is strongly inherited—If found in one identical twin, the other has a 70 percent chance of also having the disease.

Some Background

To understand PCOS, let's first look at normal hormone balance. There are two areas in your brain that are vital to normal menstrual function and monthly cycles resulting in ovulation:

1. Your hypothalamus produces GnRH (gonadotropin-releasing hormone).
2. In response to GnRH, your pituitary produces FSH to stimulate your egg growth in the ovary and estradiol (estrogen), and LH to signal ovulation and progesterone production.

GnRH tells your pituitary to send an appropriate balance of FSH and LH to the ovary, stimulating both male (androgen) and female (estrogen and progesterone) hormone production, as well as ovulation. Prior to ovulation, FSH and estrogen (from the growing egg inside an ovarian follicle cyst) are the dominant hormones, but following ovulation, LH and progesterone are dominant. (Progesterone prepares your uterine lining [endometrium] for pregnancy.) Hormones from the ovary give feedback to your brain to keep this balance.

Now for PCOS (Using a Workplace Model)

PCOS involves a 'vicious cycle' of hormone imbalance. Hormones are simply proteins produced in one organ that affect other parts of the body, and the main players in PCOS are GnRH, FSH, LH, estradiol (the most common estrogen), progesterone, testosterone, and insulin.

In PCOS, your hypothalamus (think overbearing boss), sends continuous messages to the pituitary (think underappreciated employee), but the latter seems a bit too hypersensitive (from being underpaid) and responds by making too much LH (think spite). This hormonal chaos (due to no human resources director) prevents the hypothalamus, the pituitary, and the ovary from communicating effectively, resulting in no ovulation (time for team building activities for the workplace).

HOW TO DIAGNOSE PCOS

To diagnose PCOS, we use the following clinical guidelines from the Rotterdam consensus conference in 2003, and you need to meet two out of the three criteria:

1. Ovulation dysfunction (menstrual intervals of more than 35 days, or fewer than 8 menses per year) or lack of ovulation (Of note: Regular monthly menstrual cycles cannot ensure you ovulate, so blood testing is necessary to confirm.)

2. Elevated blood levels of androgens (testosterone) or the physical exam shows hirsutism (unwanted dark hair in male pattern areas: upper lip, chin, sideburn, neck, chest, lower midline of abdomen, upper inner thighs, lower back, and upper back).

3. Classic "string of pearls" appearance on pelvic ultrasound of the ovaries—20 or more small normal cysts (antral follicles) seen in either ovary

NOTE: Before your doctor makes the diagnosis of PCOS, other diseases that can cause ovulation dysfunction or elevated androgens must be excluded, such as thyroid disease, elevated prolactin, and adrenal disorders.

THE SIX SIGNS AND SYMPTOMS OF PCOS

1. Reproductive (irregular menstrual cycles, hirsutism, infertility, and pregnancy complications)—A chronic lack of ovulation results in the lining of the uterus (endometrium) having a disorderly buildup and overgrowth. Breakthrough bleeding and even continuous bleeding occurs that can result in anemia (think if you put a hose in your pool and forgot to turn it off; that's analogous to the vaginal bleeding in PCOS, i.e., overflow). The BCP is usually very effective at controlling bleeding as well as reducing the effects of hirsutism. A consequence of elevated androgens that results in ovulation dysfunction, hirsutism can be seen in up to 70 percent of you who have PCOS. Due to ovulation dysfunction, infertility occurs and is treated with medication to induce ovulation. A one-time surgery called *ovarian drilling* has often been used to successfully induce and maintain monthly ovulation. Pregnancy complications from PCOS include miscarriage, diabetes, and high blood pressure; the latter two are higher in obese patients.

2. Psychological (anxiety, depression, body image)—We, as health professionals, must be vigilant regarding the psychological consequences of PCOS. Given the higher risk of anxiety and depression with PCOS, clinicians should provide you with tools to work through the emotional toll of this disease. Helpful strategies include mild to moderate exercise, yoga, meditation, and acupuncture. You may also benefit from speaking with a reproductive health counselor.

3. Weight—While there is no consensus on the diet to manage PCOS, there is clear agreement on the need for an appropriate BMI. Almost all the complications of PCOS can be improved with lifestyle and behavior modification toward a normal BMI. Regular follow up with a goal-oriented program can be valuable. As little as a 5 to 10 percent weight loss will help you improve ovulation.

3. Obstructive sleep apnea (OSA)—Common in PCOS women who are obese, OSA can have significant effects on quality of life. Clinicians must be knowledgeable of the signs and symptoms. The diagnosis is helped by screening questions, followed by referral to a specialist as indicated. Easy screening tool options are STOP-BANG (SB), Epworth Sleepiness Scale (ESS), and the 4-Variable screening tool (4-V).

5. Endometrial precancer—There is a twofold to sixfold increased risk of endometrial cancer due to lack of progesterone from ovulation dysfunction allowing estrogen buildup to the lining of the uterus (endometrium), which results in a progression from normal lining to hyperplasia to precancer to cancer. Signs of concern are menstrual intervals greater than 90 days and/or an endometrium measuring more than 7 millimeters (0.3 inches) on ultrasound. Women often present with abnormal bleeding. Treatment begins with progesterone but can involve a hysterectomy in extreme cases.

6. Metabolic Syndrome occurs in nearly 40 percent of PCOS patients (twice as high as the general population). The more hirsutism you experience, the more likely you will have Metabolic Syndrome, defined as having three or more of the following risk factors:

    a. Insulin resistance (IR) or prediabetes—Defined as an abnormal two-hour glucose tolerance test; alternative testing may include fasting glucose and insulin or hemoglobin A1c

    b. Obesity—Defined as a BMI greater than 30 and/or waist circumference ≥ 88 centimeters (34.6 inches) in women

    c. High blood pressure—Elevated systolic and/or diastolic blood pressure of ≥130/85 mmHg

    d. Elevated triglycerides—Elevated fasting serum triglycerides ≥ 150 mg/dL

    e. Elevated cholesterol—Fasting high-density lipoprotein (HDL) cholesterol < 50 Mg/dL

Carly was diagnosed with PCOS in 2012, when she was 33. She and her husband, Robert, had decided it was time to start a family, so she stopped taking BCPs following seven consecutive years of use. Instead of pregnancy, her body started waging war on her. "I gained an alarming amount of weight and had acne," Carly said. "I suffered a miscarriage and was told by my then doctor that I just needed to lose weight. I just wish more people knew that PCOS is so much more than something that can be cured by losing weight. I wish more people that are affected by this disease would understand that they are not alone."

How Do You Manage PCOS?

Prior to pregnancy, we always address the medical risks of PCOS, as seen in this table:

MEDICAL RISKS OF PCOS	
Prediabetes/Diabetes	Hirsutism
Elevated blood pressure	Uterine cancer
Elevated cholesterol/triglycerides	Anxiety/depression
Elevated BMI	Obstructive sleep apnea

Following appropriate treatment of Metabolic Syndrome, it's time to address the reproductive issues of PCOS. If pregnancy is not desired, then you can take BCPs to control hormonal imbalance, unless you have a medical contraindication—if so, a progesterone-like hormone can be provided to provide regular menstrual flow to protect the lining of the uterus (endometrium) from unopposed estrogen stimulation and the risk of uterine cancer.

ADVANTAGES OF BCPS
- Regulates menstrual cycle bleeding
- Reduces hirsutism
- Reduces ovarian and uterine cancer
- Controls ovarian cyst formation

CONTRAINDICATIONS TO BCPS
- History of venous thromboembolism (blood clot)
- History of stroke and heart attack
- Uncontrolled high blood pressure
- Cigarette smoking ≥ 15 per day in women ≥ 35 years of age

Ovulation Induction

While clomiphene citrate is the oldest oral fertility medication to induce ovulation, recent recommendations support letrozole for first line usage, particularly in women whose BMI is greater than 30. Both clomiphene and letrozole trick the brain, in different ways, to reduce the amount of estrogen your brain sees, thereby increasing FSH stimulation to the ovary in anticipation of follicle cyst development of a mature egg. Pregnancy success is based on the patient's age and body weight, that is, the lower BMI and age, the higher the success.

The next step to induce ovulation, if oral medication is not successful, are the options of taking injectable medication (gonadotropins) or undergoing LOD.

GONADOTROPIN INJECTABLE MEDS	
Pros	**Cons**
Noninvasive	Expensive medications
Recurrent attempts at ovulation each month	Risk of ovarian hyperstimulation
Less expensive than IVF	Risk of multiple births

LAPAROSCOPIC OVARIAN DRILLING	
Pros	**Cons**
One-time procedure	Surgical complications (rare)
May result in years of natural ovulation	Lack of guarantee for ovulation
Natural risk of multiple birth	Risk of ovarian failure (rare)
Usually covered by insurance	Not needed if pursuing IVF

Gonadotropins are expensive and not often covered by insurance, unless you live in a mandated infertility insurance state or country. The major risk of these medications are high order multiple births because there is no control over how many ovarian follicles develop and release eggs, how many eggs fertilize to become embryos, and how many embryos implant in the uterus. This explains the misunderstood risk of high order multiple births—the risk is higher when not proceeding with IVF due to the inability to control how many embryos enter the uterine cavity from your fallopian tubes. With IVF, your physician only transfers a predetermined number of embryos that will offer you a reasonable chance of success and low risk of multiple births. The other risk of gonadotropins is ovarian hyperstimulation syndrome (OHSS), particularly in PCOS women, from excessive ovarian follicle response to the medication that can result in fluid accumulation in the abdomen, lungs, as well as potentially life-threatening blood clots. Fortunately the risk of OHSS has dramatically decreased over the last one to two decades due to alternative medications to trigger the release of the eggs after stimulation, namely, from hCG to GnRH agonist. (For more about OHSS, see chapter 16.)

With successful ovulation induction in nearly 70 percent of patients, LOD, if successful, potentially avoids a more expensive IVF cycle and allows for regular menstrual cycles, thus potentially avoiding subsequent fertility treatments and reducing the risk of endometrial hyperplasia. LOD is a well-established outpatient procedure to induce ovulation surgically, first reported in 1984.

While the exact way LOD works is not understood, the procedure involves multiple punctures into the ovary using electrocautery, resulting in a reduction in the male hormone producing (theca) cells. Pregnancy success rates are typically 50 to 80 percent. If you have a BMI ≥ 35, you are less likely to successfully respond to LOD.

LOD can restore ovulation with regular menses and has significant benefits including treating infertility, protecting the uterine lining from cancer, reducing testosterone to improve acne and unwanted hair growth, and avoiding anemia from continued abnormal uterine bleeding.

The best candidates for LOD are those of you with PCOS who have been unsuccessful on medication to ovulate and have a BMI < 35.

According to the release by ASRM and ESHRE (the European Society for Human Reproduction and Embryology) of the 2018 "International evidence-based guideline for the assessment and management of polycystic ovary syndrome," therapeutic options areas follows.

1) *Combined BCPs*: This is considered the first-line treatment for irregular menstrual cycles and bleeding as well as for hirsutism (unwanted hair growth in a male pattern from elevated male hormone levels).

2) *Metformin*: This is a diabetic medication that has been shown to improve ovulation function in PCOS patients and treat weight, hormonal, and metabolic problems, but its effect on improving the live birth rate is not clear.

3) *Inositol*: This is a natural protein that decreases the insulin resistance often seen in PCOS women, but its use needs further research.

4) *Letrozole*: Originally meant to treat breast cancer, this medication is now considered the "go-to" for ovulation induction in PCOS women, replacing clomiphene citrate.

5) *Gonadotropins* or *LOD*: When oral medication is not successful, these options should be discussed as next steps.

6) *IVF*: Following treatment attempts using oral medication and then injectable medications or surgery, IVF is the third-line therapy for ovulation dysfunction.

OTHER RECOMMENDATIONS FOR MANAGEMENT OF PCOS

1) *Excess weight*: Women should receive appropriate education for self-empowerment with the goal of encouraging healthy behaviors in the areas of proper nutrition and exercise.

2) *Depressive and anxiety symptoms*: PCOS women should be screened and given support as needed for their emotional well-being and quality of life.

In Conclusion

As in all of medicine, when treating PCOS, we proceed with the most conservative to the most aggressive treatments. After optimizing all the metabolic problems with PCOS, we start with oral medications to induce ovulation and then advance to injectable medications or surgery, and finally, to IVF. First, second, and third, a healthy lifestyle is vital and includes exercise and proper diet when TTC as well as during your pregnancy. While there is no specific diet or exercise for women with PCOS, the Mediterranean Diet (see page 30) has been shown to improve health and fertility.

CHAPTER 14

The Male Factor

A tension-breaking comment that I share with my patients at their first visit when we talk about male-factor infertility is, "the few times we will hear from or see your husband will be their calling for the results, every hour, of their sperm analysis." This is obviously a tremendous exaggeration (it's every two hours!) but it speaks to the differences between the sexes regarding your pursuit of a diagnosis. As women, you appear eager and somewhat content to find an answer and rarely experience remorse or shame if there is a female factor. Unfortunately, this is not true for men—many times you are devastated or even embarrassed if there is a male factor, particularly a severe one.

So why are you all so different in your responses to the contributing causes of your infertility? I think it comes down to outdated and, dare I say, chauvinistic mindsets. We can't argue the point that when it comes to parenteral investment during the pregnancy; women win hands down. The fact that women need to successfully have the embryo implant and then carry the baby for nine months clearly tilts the physical and biologic work of reproduction given the male's contribution is initially limited to ejaculation. And my reason for implicating chauvinism is my belief that men have a feeling of threat regarding their sexual prowess, that is, male infertility equates to a decreased masculinity.

This distinction of the male and female contribution to reproduction is, absolutely, not meant to disrespect the emotional bond of a couple and their equal sincerity in desiring a baby. Rather, it may help you all appreciate your different approaches toward the pursuit of pregnancy.

Despite 40 percent of infertility causes being due to the male partner, and 30 percent being from both male and female factors, you and even physicians may neglect the importance of the male factor. These percentages for causes of infertility are relatively constant among cultural and ethnic populations.

Fortunately, with increasing numbers of urologists undergoing specialty training in male reproduction, along with continued advances in reproductive technology, infertile men can feel encouraged.

After obtaining a complete medical history, your physician will ask you to provide an SA. The WHO, 5th edition standards released in 2010 (*2010 WHO Guidelines for Semen Analysis*), classifies a normal sperm concentration as 15 million or more sperm per milliliter, with a motility (total movement) of 40 percent or more, and morphology (normal shapes) of 4 percent or more.

NOTE: Fertility clinics that are not using this latest guideline from the WHO are potentially causing you unnecessary worry and testing. My advice is to ask your physician which WHO edition is being used to interpret your sperm analysis. Unless it's the 5th edition, you can simply ask for the report and use the above values. (Note that the sperm analysis report typically states which WHO edition is being used.)

The sperm analysis cut-off values for normal are not meant to classify fertile vs. non-fertile. Here's how they came up with the reference ranges: They studied men who had proven fertility (i.e., impregnated their partner within one year of attempts at conception).

Above the cut-off values were 95 percent of the men and below were 5 percent. Remember all were fertile. Below the cut-off values, men still contributed to a pregnancy, but there were just a lesser percentage of men who fathered a child. Traditionally, the SA correlates with sperm fertilization potential. One abnormal SA, obtained following a two- to five-day abstinence from a prior ejaculation, warrants your referral to a fellowship-trained male reproductive specialist. While some doctors and patients may believe they can defer a urology evaluation and opt for IVF with ICSI to overcome the male factor and achieve fertilization, the importance of a male examination cannot be overstated—an abnormal SA, particularly when severe, may reveal a life-threatening health issue in up to 2 percent of you.

Genetics and Your Fertility

The urology evaluation will investigate you for physical, hormonal, and genetic causes of male infertility. The physician should know your family history of infertility, medications, anabolic steroid use, environmental toxin exposure, and tobacco, alcohol, and recreational drug use. At the physical exam, the urologist will check your scrotal sac for a varicocele (see later in this chapter) and for a congenital bilateral absence of the vas deferens (CBAVD). (The vas is the tube that carries sperm from the testes to the urethra during ejaculation. It's also the tube urologists cut and partially remove when a man no longer desires fertility and has a vasectomy.) You will also have hormone testing, particularly if you have very low to no sperm in the ejaculate, including FSH, total testosterone, LH, free testosterone, estradiol, and prolactin.

Approximately 50 percent of male infertility involves genetic abnormalities. The diagnosis of infertility may not only indicate a genetic problem with you, but also could place the fertility of your offspring at risk. When you have a severe male factor and no blockage of the male ducts, your genetic testing will consist of a karyotype for complete chromosome analysis (abnormal in approximately 7 percent and more common based on the severity of the abnormal SA) and Y chromosome microdeletion (YCMD, explained in greater detail below), found in 10 to 15 percent with very low to no sperm in the ejaculate.

If you have chromosomal abnormalities, your children are at risk for genetic defects, miscarriage, and birth defects. Through a growing understanding of the genetics of male infertility, a chromosomal abnormality can be found in less than 1 percent of men with a normal SA, 5 percent of men with oligozoospermia (severe low sperm counts, i.e., less than five million per milliliter), and in 10 to 15 percent of men with azoospermia (ejaculate without sperm). Sex chromosomal errors (with the most common being Klinefelter syndrome) represent two-thirds of all chromosomal abnormalities.

Y CHROMOSOME MICRODELETION (YCMD)

Three regions of the Y-chromosome (male sex chromosome) reveal the most common YCMDs, namely AZFa, AZFb, and AZFc. If you have a YCMD, the importance of identifying the specific location is related to the prognosis of retrieving sperm using microsurgery on the testes—because only men with AZFc can have sperm potentially obtained. A trick to remember the significance of the AZF deletions is AZF "a" is awful, AZF "b" is bad, and AZF "c" is cool and can result in conception. If you are AZFa, we would not recommend trying to obtain sperm from your testes.

Treatable Causes of Male Infertility

The secondary goal of your evaluation is to determine if the infertility is treatable. The leading causes of treatable male infertility include the following.

VARICOCELE

This condition is sort of like varicose veins and refers to a congestion of blood in the veins surrounding your testes. Why is this bad? The testes, as you know, are outside the body and are very temperature sensitive; unlike the ovaries that must remain body temperature. When it's too hot out, the scrotal sac relaxes and allows the testes to fall away from the body to lower their temperature; in cold temperature, your scrotal sac draws the testes closer to your abdomen to increase to maintain their appropriate temperature. This is why you hear about the risk of too many hot tubs when TTC because the increased testicular temperature can damage the temperature-sensitive sperm.

This type of venous congestion is usually present if you are tall and occurs mostly on your left side due to testicular vein anatomy. The American Urology Association considers a varicocele as clinically significant when (1) it can be felt on clinical examination (feels like a bag of worms) as opposed to needing ultrasound to diagnose; (2) the SA is abnormal; and (3) infertility is present.

A varicocele is treatable with surgery, usually performed on an outpatient basis. Studies have had mixed results regarding the outcome of varicocelectomy (tying off the dilated veins to reduce congestion around the testes). There appears to be value in the surgery, particularly if you are young with large varicoceles and no decrease in testicular volume (TV) from prolonged venous congestion.

AZOOSPERMIA (NO SPERM IN THE EJACULATE)

During an infertility evaluation, about 10 to 15 percent of men who are deemed infertile will be told they have no sperm in their ejaculate (about 1 percent of the general population). This news is about as bad as it can get after you have been TTC and looking into the "why?" While donor sperm is always an option, and much less expensive, here are five causes for this devastating diagnosis.

1. **Retrograde ejaculation** occurs in 1 percent of infertile men, but in 15 percent of men with azoospermia. RE results from the semen being redirected into your bladder, rather than the normal path through the urethra and out the penis. How do we find this out? On a basic SA, if your volume is low with no sperm, it is reasonable to repeat

the SA, but following ejaculation, you urinate into a cup so your urine can be analyzed for sperm. RE treatment lacks a consensus, but one easy option involves pre-ejaculation medication to raise the pH of the urine for sperm to survive in the bladder. The man then voids for sperm collection followed by IUI of the washed sperm.

Causes of RE are as follows:

- Nerve damage caused by a medical condition, such as diabetes, multiple sclerosis, Parkinson's disease, or a spinal cord injury
- Surgery involving your prostate or bladder
- Certain medications to treat enlarged prostate, high blood pressure, or depression
- Radiation therapy to treat cancer in your pelvis

2. Obstructive (blocked) azoospermia (OA) may be surgically corrected to allow for natural conception attempts with ejaculated sperm. If no sperm can be ejaculated, then the alternative method of using your sperm, which is usually very successful given the reason is a blockage and not production, is a minor office procedure called TESA. Sperm obtained from your testes is immature to fertilize naturally. It would be great to use TESA sperm with IUI, but fertilization would not occur. IVF is necessary for fertilization with TESA sperm using the advanced technology of ICSI (the process of isolating and injecting a single sperm into the egg to overcome fertilization problems). Although fertilization and embryo development are slightly lower with TESA sperm as opposed to ejaculated sperm, this is an exciting option to give you hope for a biologically related baby.

A unique cause of obstruction, CBAVD has an approximate 80 percent association with you being a carrier for cystic fibrosis, and the fertility treatment also requires TESA.

3. Non-obstructive azoospermia (NOA) is the usual diagnosis if you have elevated FSH, small testes, and normal ejaculatory volume. Because NOA can be associated with genetic causes, karyotype and YCMD studies (as discussed earlier) are appropriate and may predict the likelihood of successful sperm retrieval.

4. Cryptorchidism (testis in the abdomen) is when one or both testes abnormally remain in the abdomen at birth, rather than normally descending into the appropriate location in the scrotum. Once this occurs, the male remains at risk for abnormal SA despite the surgical relocation of the testes to their normal position or even if one of the testes requires surgical removal.

Other: These next two categories are determined after hormonal testing of pituitary gonadotropins (FSH, LH) to provide information on a likely cause of your azoospermia:

- Elevated FSH/LH with low testosterone suggests testicular failure. Genetic testing of your chromosomes should occur next to provide you a reasonable prognosis for a sperm retrieval with a TESA.
- Low FSH/LH with low testosterone suggest hypothalamic disorders (such as Kallman's syndrome, which is a congenital disorder involving the inability to sexually mature); pituitary disorders; or anabolic steroid use (seen in bodybuilders or in men given testosterone supplementation for low energy or low libido—see below). Fortunately, men who are making inadequate FSH/LH can receive injectable gonadotropins (just like their female partner may need to ovulate), which is very effective to stimulate production of sperm and testosterone.

5. Vasectomy is really a subcategory of obstructive azoospermia. Physicians have long believed a vasectomy reversal is usually unsuccessful when the vasectomy was performed more than ten years prior. While the duration of time from vasectomy influences success following reversal, medical evidence reveals reversal is an option when performed by experienced surgeons and the female partner is less than 35 years old. The alternative to vasectomy reversal is IVF with ICSI using TESA (explained above).

TESTOSTERONE (T) SUPPLEMENTATION

Many urologists and family practitioners order blood testing of testosterone during your routine exam if you feel fatigue, or during a male infertility evaluation. That's not the bad part. The bad part is when they prescribe you testosterone if the blood testosterone level is low. As in bodybuilders on anabolic steroids, testosterone supplementation can suppress pituitary FSH and dramatically lower sperm production to the point of azoospermia, especially if the testosterone treatment is injections.

Blood testosterone should only be ordered as part of your infertility evaluation if the sperm analysis is repeatedly abnormal and/or you present with symptoms of testosterone deficiency. Testosterone supplementation should never be given to you if you are TTC now or in the near future due to the risk of shutting down your sperm production.

Another caveat: You also should use caution if taking testosterone due to the risk of dangerous blood clot formations.

OTHER CONCERNS

Due to potential harmful effects of electromagnetic radiation, recent multiple studies have demonstrated impaired sperm motility if you use a cell phone (and, who doesn't?). The study findings included

- Reduced sperm motility by 8 percent
- Reduced sperm viability

While there may be negative effects on sperm from cell phone usage, there is no definitive evidence for an impact on the natural live birth rate. If you are experiencing a prolonged time to conceive and/or meet the definition of infertility, I would reduce or at least be conscious of the duration of your cell phone use.

FERTILITY HEALTH RECOMMENDATIONS—LIFESTYLES TO AVOID

- Avoid tobacco (may cause genetic alterations of sperm and affect the female partner through second-hand smoke).
- Avoid recreational drug use.
- Avoid excessive alcohol.
- Avoid bodybuilding hormones or testosterone.
- Avoid prolonged elevation of scrotal temperature (to prevent impaired sperm production).
- Avoid STIs.

In Conclusion

Today, more options exist that were unavailable until recently and even in cases of severe male-factor infertility, pregnancy may still be achieved. However, due to the shared nature of the decision-making process between your physician and you, it is vital for you and your female partner to have a complete fertility evaluation and an open dialogue with your fertility doctor.

If you are a couple experiencing infertility, you must remember that male problems may be the sole or contributing reason for the couple's failure to conceive about half of the time. Male problems are best evaluated and treated by a reproductive urology specialist. Using a proactive approach, you can avoid missed opportunities for a potential diagnosis and receive the timeliest and most efficient pathway to start or expand your family.

CHAPTER 15
Self-Help Fertility Methods

pproximately 85 percent of couples where the woman is less than age 35 conceive within one year of conception attempts. When the cause of infertility is unexplained, about 60 percent of couples will conceive over the following 3 to 5 years. Clearly, some couples just take longer to conceive—a fact not well received by many of you struggling to have a child. Nevertheless, natural attempts at conception for at least the appropriate duration (based on the woman's age) should be maximized unless the couple have risk factors that would interfere with and/or prevent conception. As presented in the chapter on "Confronting Infertility," in 2009 the WHO and the International Committee for Monitoring Assisted Reproductive defined infertility as "a disease of the reproductive system defined by the failure to achieve a clinical pregnancy after 12 months or more of regular unprotected sexual intercourse." While agreeing with this definition, the ASRM, in 2013, supported an "earlier evaluation and treatment may be justified based on medical history and physical findings and is warranted after 6 months for women over age 35 years."

"Why can't I just do this naturally?"

The lament from many heterosexual patients is the disappointment over your inability for a natural conception. Of all the diseases in medicine, infertility appears to be unique in that many of you beat your chest and long to "heal thyself" rather than receive assistance with fertility treatment. Don't get me wrong—I understand the attraction of conceiving privately through intimacy rather than through a procedure in a medical office around strangers! And I believe fertility physicians should do all they can to optimize your ability to conceive naturally or with the least physical and financial investment. But I simply do not understand the initial enthusiasm for a child followed by the tacit but reluctant acceptance of childlessness rather than proceeding with fertility care (as long as it's affordable).

In my 20 years as a fertility specialist, I have rarely met a woman, man, or couple whom I believed were not prepared to parent. Most of you who come to a fertility clinic have put your heart and soul into choosing to parent and are willing to undergo all the "poking and prodding" we prescribe for an answer. But a low percentage of you will avoid fertility treatment options because "it wasn't meant to be."

"God's Will"

My intention here is not to offend anyone, but I'm a staunch critic of the opinion that the reason for your infertility and lack of a child is due to "God's will." Perhaps I am too simplistic, but I do not believe a higher power would intervene to prevent you from fulfilling an innate and profound desire originating from and resulting in love. This just seems so maleficent as well as unfair to you, your partner, and your potential future child.

Medicine has allowed so many diseases to be successfully treated, why not infertility? If there is no harm to you and medical evidence supports its use, I fully embrace pursuing all methods of curing disease, including infertility. What's unclear to me is why some of you resist embracing advances in reproductive medicine, outside of moral or religious objections. Some of you may view the use of fertility treatment options as a failure of your journey to a baby. But there is nothing further from the truth! My advice is to change "God's will" to "Thank God" there is such advanced fertility treatment that might bring your baby home.

Over the Counter

Natural remedies are all the rage in health care. Vitamins, herbs, acupuncture, and any natural supplement are often the first line of approach from patients with any medical problem. Let's take acupuncture, for example. Over 10 years ago, medical studies were suggesting acupuncture improved fertility. That's all it took; soon thereafter, the fertility industry was inundated by acupuncture specialists advertising their fertility prowess while patients flocked to their door. This is not to disparage the field of acupuncture—I have partnered with wonderful Oriental Medical Doctors (OMDs) and my patients and I love this service. We included our OMD for more than five years until new medical evidence convincingly refuted the original claims. What we now know is that some, though not all studies show support for the use of acupuncture to improve the live birth rate with IVF—perhaps timing and type of acupuncture plays a more important role. There is more convincing evidence on the benefits of acupuncture in stress reduction.

You Are Not Defined by Your Ability to Conceive Naturally

I believe we were all chosen to be someone special and unique. So, why do some of you have as much disappointment toward undergoing fertility treatment as you do toward your disease—because many of you view treatment as representing failure of your plan for the way it was meant to happen.

In over 20 years of talking to infertility patients just like you, I have yet to meet anyone—and I mean anyone—whose life is exactly as they planned it! It just doesn't happen that way. Nevertheless, I believe we are defined by how we overcome adversity and maximize the success of our life irrespective of the bumps and bruises along the way. The ability to procreate is not a talent or a skill to boast. Rather, how we parent, contribute to our world, and/or bounce back from adversity are the characteristics to awe.

When to Immediately See a Fertility Specialist

While there are over-the-counter/natural products that claim to treat infertility, most, if not all, causes of true infertility (as defined above) are not amenable to natural cures with the exceptions of optimizing your BMI from the extremes of body weight for women and obesity for men; and smoking cessation for the couple. On the next page are nine problems that warrant your seeking direct care by an infertility specialist.

WOMEN

1. Very irregular periods or none at all
2. History of tubal ligation (tubes tied)
3. Congenital absence of a uterus or one that was surgically removed

MEN

1. Vasectomy
2. Unable to ejaculate or release any semen
3. OTC sperm test shows no sperm

COUPLE

1. Carriers for the same genetic disorder or have a significant genetic inheritable disease
2. Newly diagnosed with cancer and interested in fertility preservation before cancer treatment
3. Experiencing infertility while your prior paternity has been able to conceive with someone else

I recently met a heterosexual couple (let's call them Brian and Kelly), both in their early 30s, TTC for nine months without success. They had no predisposing factors for infertility and had convinced the woman's OB/GYN to prescribe a fertility evaluation consisting of an HSG and a sperm analysis. The couple were referred to me only to obtain both tests at my clinic. The HSG (explained in chapter 5: Treatments You Should Avoid) showed only one tube was patent, allowing contrast dye to flow from the cervix into the uterus and completely through the entire tube then spill out into the pelvis. The sperm analysis showed several minor abnormalities, such as mild low morphology (the percentage of normal shaped sperm). They then returned to their OB/GYN who prescribed Kelly clomiphene citrate for three months—yet still no pregnancy. They were extremely frustrated and getting desperate.

At their first visit with me, they requested more aggressive fertility treatment. I shared my opinion that their OB/GYN ordered a fertility evaluation earlier than recommended. At the woman's age, they should try one year of conception attempts prior to consideration of a fertility evaluation. The testing results showed some abnormalities; yet, were the abnormalities so severe as to prevent conception? The answer was, unequivocally, no.

The HSG showed one opened tube; reproduction requires at least one patent fallopian tube. The sperm analysis revealed several abnormalities that suggest decreased fertilization potential but not sterility. The only true outcome from all this premature testing was anxiety in the couple.

My job was obvious but difficult—to recommend resuming natural attempts at conception, for a total of one year, using an over-the-counter OPK along with appropriately timed intercourse. While some may interpret my advice as paternalistic or unsympathetic, I reply, "Nay, nay!" My obligation is to offer evidence-based medical care, beginning with the most conservative and least costly treatment. Since the odds were still in their favor to conceive, they agreed with me. Well, over the next few months, they conceived naturally and were grateful for my recommendation because it reduced their expense and anxiety. In medicine, it is equally important to know when to treat and when not to intervene.

Optimizing Your Fertility

Given the innate motivation toward natural conception, let's review my three most important factors in conceiving:

1. AGE

The single most important factor we use to predict a woman's your monthly ability to conceive (fecundity) through natural means or by treatment is age. Your fertility begins to slowly but steadily decline beginning at age 30, with a more accelerated drop during your late 30s and into your 40s. Today more of you are deferring childbearing due to schooling, career, or personal reasons (often not finding the right partner). By waiting to have a child after age 30, you will most likely face an increasing challenge.

What are the options regarding age and fertility? The easiest answer is to begin building your family before age 30. However, this is not always practical or desirable for the reasons outlined above. Unless your personal timetable allows you to begin having children before the age of 30, you are faced with a statistically more difficult time to pregnancy unless you consider preserving your fertility with egg freezing. (For a discussion of egg freezing, see chapter 22: Preserving Fertility from Cancer.) Obviously this is a personal decision and there is no guarantee of either option being successful. Your OB/GYN or REI specialist are valuable resources to discuss this further.

While many of you know that a woman's age will directly impact her ability to procreate, fewer are aware of the consequences of advanced paternal age. (See chapter 8: Optimizing Men's Prenatal Health.) More evidence is indicating that men above age 40 experience declining fertility, increasing pregnancy loss and preterm delivery, and higher risks of children with birth defects, autism, and schizophrenia.

Bottom Line: Women should begin TTC before age 30 and men before age 40. If this schedule conflicts with your timetable, then consider egg freezing and/or sperm freezing.

2. OVULATION

To keep it simple, you should use an inexpensive over-the-counter OPK. The OPK detects, in the urine, the surge of LH produced from the region of the brain called the pituitary gland. This surge in LH results in three critical steps: (1) to release the egg; (2) to stimulate the production of progesterone (which prepares the lining of the uterus (endometrium) for embryo implantation); and (3) triggering a biologic change in the egg (maturation) enabling it to be fertilized.

All the tests for ovulation are not conclusive and only *presume* an egg is being released from your ovary. **Quiz time!** What's the only definitive proof you ovulated? A pregnancy! This may appear to be a trick question, but all the other tests for ovulation only presume the egg was released. Let's look at all the symptoms and signs consistent with ovulation:

- OPK for the LH surge
- Cervical mucus becomes watery and stretchy (called Spinnbarkeit) due to high levels of estrogen right before ovulation. Right after ovulation, the mucus thickens to reduce infection and prevent entry of additional sperm from potentially fertilizing another egg.
- Lower abdominal cramping (called Mittleschmerz) from swelling of the capsule just prior to ovulation
- BBT resulting in a 0.5 Fahrenheit (0.3 Celsius) degree rise in your temperature, to usually above 98 degrees Fahrenheit (36.7 degrees Celsius) at ovulation due to progesterone elevation. (See chapter 16: Understanding Ovulation.)
- Endometrial biopsy involves a minor office procedure that samples examines the uterine lining to determine if the glands and stroma of the lining have developed appropriately to optimize embryo implantation.

Bottom Line: If your cycles are regular and monthly (typically 28 to 30-day intervals) along with ovulatory signs, then this is good evidence you are ovulating.

3. TIMING OF INTERCOURSE

"How often and when should we have sex?" Boy oh boy, if had a dime for every time a patient has asked me this question! Ah, but to dream. I don't recall ever mentioning to an infertility couple, "You are having too much sex, slow down!" This is not because most of you abstain from sex or because you lack intimacy, but because you have been guided on how often to have sex from all the FMDs you know. FMDs? Yes, you know, Fertile Myrtle Doctors. Who are they? Well, they just so happen to be the premier authority on procreation. Why? Because they had a baby naturally, silly! Don't you get it? As long as someone has experienced the miracle of conception and childbirth, they often—erroneously—believe they have received a doctorate in reproductive biology and are able to advise *anyone* who is TTC. And, to think, I wasted 14 years of training!

Let's look at the reality of the matter. Fertile times for a woman occur six days prior and up to the day of ovulation, so I advise you have frequent sexual relations during this time, about every day to every other day. However, the time during your cycle that will result in maximum fertility is over the three-day period up to and including the day of ovulation, that is, from one day prior through one day after a positive OPK result. It should be noted there is no medical evidence for improved fertility based on intercourse position, time of day, female orgasm, or you remaining flat for a prolonged time following your partner's ejaculation.

Most commercial-based vaginal lubricants will decrease sperm motility and therefore can lower the chance of a pregnancy. However, lubricants such as mineral oil, canola oil, Pre-Seed (INGfertility), and ConceivEase (Reproductive Laboratory) do not appear to have a negative effect on sperm function.

Bottom Line: Optimal fertility occurs with an increase of intercourse over the period of three days prior to, and including, ovulation.

In Conclusion

The more you are aware of your body, optimal times to conceive, and factors that will increase or decrease your chance for conception, the less anxiety you may feel. Most importantly, by maximizing your understanding and utilization of this chapter's recommendations, you may (hopefully) avoid having to see a fertility specialist!

CHAPTER 16

Fertility Medications

"Wow, that medicine's great!" said no patient in history. The field of infertility is no exception and you are no less vulnerable than patients in other fields. A chapter on medicines may usually be boring, but I'm going to do my best prevent that from happening!

Just like these medicines are a necessity, so is the explanation of these medicines in an infertility book. Since this is a book on infertility, let's try to make this section more appealing by answering the Who, What, Where, When, How, and Why about reproductive drugs to conceive.

Who?

For those of you TTC, there are two categories of women who use fertility drugs, each with a different goal:

- Ovulatory—To increase the number of eggs released by ovulation from two to as high as four
- Anovulatory—To overcome a lack of ovulation by helping you release one or two eggs

Fertility drugs for women originally gained FDA approval to help women who did not ovulate, hence the prevailing term for treatment cycles, "ovulation induction." As time passed, it became clear, these drugs also were able to increase the number of eggs an ovulatory woman will release.

When you go to your fertility doctor, these drugs will be the first line treatment.

What?

OVULATION INDUCERS

- **Oral:** Of all the reasons for not ovulating, you can only use oral fertility medications for PCOS (see chapter 13). This is because this category drug requires your brain to be communicating effectively between the hypothalamus and pituitary. The general way these drugs work is to trick the brain into thinking there is not enough estradiol (estrogen) around, so the brain goes into overdrive to increase stimulation to the ovary. Two global drug names are clomiphene citrate (FDA approved in the United States for ovulation), which works directly on the brain receptors, and letrozole (not FDA approved for ovulation induction in the United States), which reduces estradiol production by blocking the enzyme called aromatase. Both mechanisms increase signals by the pituitary's FSH to stimulate the ovaries.

- **Injectable:** The drugs that make you feel like a "pincushion" during your stimulation cycle—gonadotropins are a type of ovulation-induction medication that are the natural hormones FSH and LH. These are known as human menopausal gonadotropin (FSH/LH) and follitropin (FSH), and they are used to stimulate the ovaries to produce many dominant follicles (large simple ovarian cysts with eggs ready to ovulate and be fertilized) by overriding the natural cycle that only produces one egg each month. Gonadotropins are currently administered by injection and are typically used in IVF cycles.

These fertility medications can be used in combination with IUI or IVF to enhance your chance for conception.

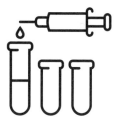

OVULATION BLOCKERS

- **GnRH Agonist:** During the early days of IVF in the 1980s, we did not have medicine to stop you from prematurely ovulating during stimulation. The downside—this medication required daily injections up to two weeks to take effect prior to stimulation, which means more days of shots for you!

- **GnRH Antagonist:** At the start of the 21st century, GnRH antagonist medication entered IVF and the beauty of this medication was it was equally effective as GnRH agonist while allowing administration in the middle of stimulation, which means fewer shots for you! Today, GnRH antagonist protocols have replaced agonist cycles as the standard stimulation protocol.

TRIGGERS FOR MATURING AND OVULATING THE EGG

- **hCG:** For decades, following the appropriate number of days of ovarian stimulation for IUI or IVF, the standard way to mature eggs prior to ovulation or egg retrieval was the injection of hCG. This injection used to be intramuscular and then changed to subcutaneous (like all the other injectable fertility medications). It works because it is structurally very similar to your body's LH that naturally signals ovulation. Ironically, this is the hormone of pregnancy, and its testing is the basis for home pregnancy tests. If you have received hCG to ovulate, your home pregnancy test will turn positive for about a week.

- **GnRH agonist:** After the GnRH antagonist came into vogue, researchers began looking at ways to reduce the risk of a dangerous side effect to stimulation, namely OHSS. The major culprit that triggers OHSS is hCG; if we could replace hCG, then IVF would be even less risky.

Well, if the body uses LH to naturally ovulate, why not use LH? Because the LH does not last long enough when administered and would require very large amounts for a patient. The solution? Give what triggers LH, namely, GnRH in the form of the agonist by stimulating the pituitary to release its own LH.

- **Advantage:** Dramatic reduction in OHSS
- **Disadvantage:** Not as effective to support the lining of the uterus after egg retrieval. This is ideal for a patient at risk of OHSS and will not undergo a fresh embryo transfer, but will have all the eggs or embryos frozen.

Where?

The "where" is your doctor's office. Traditionally, a patient visits a physician in their office who prescribes medications as indicated. Fast forward to the 21st century and you will find a plethora of over-the-counter, formerly prescription medications. For our purposes, fertility medications require a prescription. However, there is a growing trend, and concern, of obtaining medications from prescription-free websites. While this may be convenient, less expensive, and somewhat empowering for some patients, the risks far outweigh any benefit. Without being advised and monitored by your physician, women on fertility medications can be unaware they're producing an excessive number of ovarian follicles that can risk multiple births (and not just twins!) as well as OHSS (see below). The problem of all unregulated prescription drugs available through online pharmacies prompted the U.S. FDA, to release the following warnings to patients about these medications in 2016:

- They might be fake, contaminated, ineffective, or otherwise unsafe.
- They have not been evaluated by FDA for safety and efficacy.
- They may not contain the appropriate amount of active ingredients.
- They may contain harmful ingredients.

Here's more from the FDA to help you know if your pharmacy is safe:

- Requires a valid prescription
- Provides a physical address in the United States
- Is licensed by the state board of pharmacy in your state and the state where the pharmacy is operating
- Has a state-licensed pharmacist to answer your question

I recommend avoiding any online pharmacy that does not meet the above standards of the FDA and to have your fertility clinic advise where to obtain your medications.

When?

Fertility treatment cycles have two starting times: on your period or random.

1. Period stimulation start—This has been the traditional start day for decades in the infertility field. Your period, if you have monthly regular cycles, assures us you are not pregnant at the beginning of the stimulation and, we believed, allows for a better stimulation of follicles.

2. Random stimulation start—There are two kinds of patients that benefit from beginning stimulation unrelated to their period:

- Cancer patients desiring fertility preservation—Because the impending cancer treatment may not allow us to wait for your period, we now start stimulation randomly in your cycle to expedite the time to egg freezing. Studies have shown a random start has no negative impact on retrieving the number of expected eggs compared with women of the same ovarian age.
- PCOS patients—Because of ovulation dysfunction, if you have PCOS, we have no way to know when, or if, your period will start. We use ultrasound (to check ovarian cysts) and blood progesterone (to check if you ovulated) to know when to start a cycle.

How?

We typically prescribe fertility oral medications for 5 days; however, there are studies that support a longer duration for those of you that do not ovulate. As for injectable medication, the duration of time you will be on the medication depends upon the time it takes for your ovaries to respond to stimulation. The average for IVF is 10 days.

Why?

Earlier we outlined the two types of patients that receive medication: those who do not ovulate naturally and those who have unexplained infertility.

What Are the Risks of Fertility Medications?

The use of fertility medications carries unique risks that vary depending on your diagnosis and your response to them. In general the most common risks, which are more often associated with the gonadotropin class drugs, include the following:

OVARIAN HYPERSTIMULATION SYNDROME (OHSS)

- **The Good News**—We rarely see this any longer because it was associated with hCG trigger and we mostly use GnRH agonist trigger if we suspect you are at risk for OHSS.
- **The Bad News**—If you get OHSS, it's uncomfortable and although rare, could get serious.
- **Multiple Births:** Since fertility medications cause more follicles to be stimulated for growth, a higher percentage of multiple births result. The multiple birth rate with clomiphene citrate or letrozole is less than 5 percent and with gonadotropins it is 15 to 20 percent per pregnancy. In order to put these statistics in perspective, the chance for you to have a multiple birth naturally is about 1 to 2 percent.
- **Ectopic Pregnancy:** This situation results when the embryo implants outside the uterus (at least 90 percent occur in one of the fallopian tubes). Ectopic pregnancy occurs in approximately 2 percent of you attempting to conceive naturally, but this number may be slightly higher with the use of fertility medications. (See chapter 17: Reproductive Procedures.)

- **Ovarian Torsion:** Twisting (torsion) of your stimulated, enlarged ovary (usually just one) can occur in about 1 percent of treatment cycles. The ovary is cut off from its blood supply, causing abdominal pain. Surgery may be required to untwist the ovary or, rarely, remove it.
- **Ovarian Cancer:** Past studies have associated fertility medications with ovarian cancer. The risk is probably more related to continued ovulation in infertility patients than medication exposure and I believe the medical evidence is reassuring. Pregnancy and the use of BCPs, both of which prevent ovulation, decrease the risk. Many more recent studies have not demonstrated a relationship between fertility drugs and ovarian cancer.

RISK FACTORS FOR OHSS

At Start of Cycle	At Time of hCG Trigger
Young age (< 33 years of age)	High number of follicles (> 25)
High AMH (> 3.4 ng/mL)	High estradiol level (> 3500 pg/mL)
History of OHSS	High egg-retrieval number (> 24)
Polycystic appearing ovaries on ultrasound	Pregnancy

OHSS occurs in about 1 to 5 percent of cycles (see table above). What happens? Your ovaries become enlarged due to overstimulation by fertility medications. The blood vessels supplying the ovaries become "leaky" and this results in fluid collecting in the abdomen. In severe cases (less than 1 percent of treatment cycles), hospitalization is required for close monitoring. The problem lasts for one to two weeks, but can be longer and more serious, if you get pregnant during that cycle. With early detection and treatment, OHSS is rarely severe and usually can be dealt with at home.

How to Reduce Fertility Drug Side Effects and Risks

Although you can't completely avoid all side effects, there are some steps to take that will reduce their chance of occurring.

- Your doctor should start you with the lowest effective dose. High doses may reduce egg quality.
- Cancel your IUI cycle if a high number of follicles develop, that is, according to ASRM guidelines, "when three or more mature follicles (> 16 to 17 mm [> 0.6 inches]) or large numbers of intermediate-sized follicles (10 to 15 mm [0.4 to 0.6 inches]) are observed" to reduce your risk of a high order multiple pregnancy.
- Use a GnRH agonist trigger if at risk for OHSS.
- Follow the ASRM guidelines of limiting the number of embryos to transfer, including elective single embryo transfer when appropriate.

Beware of fertility clinics that are overly aggressive in their treatment of infertility. Although it may initially feel good to have a doctor promising you quick success and starting with the "strongest" treatments first, you may end up with a higher chance of risk and expense.

In Conclusion

Fertility stimulation medications were originally only approved for ovulation induction. Over the years, their indication, purity, ease of administration, and risks have been refined. Their high price and side effects remain constant, but the latter has been reduced to increased awareness and enhanced monitoring along with combining their use with newer medications to reduce risks such as OHSS. The ideal injectable ovarian stimulating medication that has minimal to no risk and much lower cost has yet to arrive.

CHAPTER 17

Reproductive Procedures

As a subspecialty of OB/GYN, the field of reproductive medicine is a surgical specialty. While I love office consultations to determine the cause of your problem through a good interview, physical exam, and laboratory testing, my field is heavily weighted with procedures—some we can perform simply in the office with you awake, while others require some form of anesthetic sedation. Ultimately any recommended procedure must be supported by medical evidence with the intention of improving your outcome to have a baby.

Intrauterine Insemination (IUI)

IUI is a procedure that can be performed in your natural cycle (without fertility medication) or as part of an ovarian stimulation cycle using fertility medication. Either cycle is meant to optimize the time for the sperm and egg to meet. During a natural cycle, you can determine impending ovulation using an over-the-counter OPK. When the test line matches your line, you typically will ovulate within 24 to 36 hours. IUI can be performed that day or the next day (there is no agreement in the medical literature for the best day). If your cycle was stimulated by medication, a trigger injection (usually hCG) mimics your natural LH surge to initiate the events of ovulation. Approximately 40 to 44 hours following the trigger, the egg will release from the ovary and survive up to 24 hours. Whereas sperm can survive in the female reproductive tract up to three days, we typically time IUI 24 to 36 hours from the trigger to ensure adequate sperm are available prior to ovulation.

IUI relies on the use of fertility medications increase a woman's chances of releasing more than one egg. Fertility medication can be used to develop a single follicular cyst (follicle) on the ovary for ovulation for those of you who do not ovulate naturally or more than the usual one follicle per month in those of you who ovulate so that an increased number of eggs are exposed to sperm, thereby increasing the chances for pregnancy.

Prior to IUI, your partner's sperm (or donor sperm) are washed and concentrated into a small volume. (Placing unwashed sperm directly into the uterus can cause severe uterine cramping similar to labor pains.) The laboratory preparation of sperm selects the most active ones that are more capable of fertilizing an egg. IUI is an office procedure that places sperm via a small catheter directly into your uterus near the time when you are ovulating. A large concentration of sperm is deposited into the upper uterine cavity so the sperm are closer to the fallopian tubes, where they travel to fertilize an egg. Most women experience little or no discomfort during an IUI.

Two considerations for you with IUI:

- Sperm sorting—In the lab, we can separate the sperm sample because X and Y bearing sperm have different molecular weights. Sperm sorting can be offered to you to increase the odds of conceiving the desired sex of you baby. With a pregnancy, the likelihood of successfully sorting for sex is 85 to 90%.
- Donor sperm can used if the male partner is
  — Sterile
  — Has an extremely low sperm count
  — Carries a risk of genetic disease
  — Not applicable (i.e., you are single or a lesbian)

In Vitro Fertilization (IVF)

IVF is the assisted reproduction technology (ART) that revolutionized the fertility treatment of women following the first baby born from this process in 1978. During an IVF cycle, we stimulate your ovaries for approximately ten days to produce multiple follicles. Once the size of your dominant (or preovulatory) follicles are appropriate, you are instructed for the time of your trigger injection. Your egg retrieval is a minor procedure performed in an office-based surgery center or hospital and involves administering intravenous conscious sedation while ultrasound is used to guide a needle through your vagina into each of your ovaries to puncture the follicular cysts (follicles) and then aspirate the fluid and collect the eggs. This procedure takes less than 30 minutes and you may return to work the next day. In the lab, the eggs are immediately analyzed then inseminated later that day in anticipation of fertilization.

If you are scheduled for an embryo transfer in the same treatment cycle following your egg retrieval (called a "fresh" transfer), this is usually performed on day 3 or day 5 after egg retrieval; otherwise, the embryos are frozen for a subsequent frozen embryo transfer (FET) cycle.

An embryo transfer is a simple procedure performed while you are fully awake. Although not all clinics accommodate their patients, we always allow your partner or the person of your choice in the room—sometimes even grandmas! A speculum is placed in your vagina and your cervix is cleansed with physiologic fluid to remove mucus that could impair the transfer. The embryo is then loaded into the catheter by the embryologist, usually in the adjoining laboratory next to the procedure room and handed to your physician who places the catheter into your uterus. All clinics presumably use abdominal ultrasound guidance to position the catheter into the uterine cavity. We uniquely use TUVS because it provides a much clearer view of your uterus and you don't need a full bladder, which can very uncomfortable. Using ultrasound, we place the embryos approximately 1.5 centimeters (0.6 inches) from the top of the uterine cavity (fundus). The catheter is then handed back to the embryologist to ensure no embryo is left in the catheter. If so, we would repeat the transfer. Patients rarely have any sensation of the catheter placement and can resume all normal activity immediately following the procedure.

Of note: Bedrest is not encouraged following embryo transfer and may reduce the chance for a pregnancy.

Originally developed to assist women with damaged fallopian tubes, IVF has now emerged as the highest monthly chance for a successful pregnancy above all other treatment options, regardless of diagnosis.

IVF treatment can help couples who display the following:

- Low to no sperm in the ejaculate
- Advanced endometriosis with damage to the uterus or fallopian tubes
- Ovulation irregularities
- Female absence of or tried fallopian tube
- Unexplained reproductive issues

Primarily, there are a couple of ways to increase the success of your IVF investment. The first is reducing the use of gonadotropins (a stimulating medication) to reduce negative effects on egg quality—less is more! (See chapter 16: Fertility Medications.) Also, while there is little to no difference in success rates with using fresh versus frozen embryos, FETs reduce the risk of OHSS (see page 134). A frozen transfer has superior pregnancy rates if you responded vigorously to injectable stimulation during your fresh cycle especially if you have PCOS. Why? The endometrium is as not as receptive to an embryo in a fresh cycle when there are high levels of estradiol, apparently having a negative impact on the implantation proteins.

If you are under 38, single-embryo transfer will reduce the complications of multiple pregnancy. Choosing to undergo preimplantation genetic screening may decrease the time to pregnancy and reduce the miscarriage rate (more on this in chapter 19: Embryo Testing and Genetics).

I believe that ovarian aging should not be used to exclude you from IVF. However, older women will experience a higher percentage of embryos that are chromosomally abnormal when tested following an IVF cycle. Ovarian aging results in fewer eggs retrieved that will significantly limit the percentage of normal embryos available for transfer.

Reproductive Surgery

Based on your individual situation, reproductive surgery can treat blocked fallopian tubes, remove endometriosis, remove fibroids, repair other abnormalities of your uterus, or correct other pelvic conditions that would impair your fertility, including those involving the ovary.

For men, reproductive surgery may help alleviate conditions such as varicocele (varicose veins of the testes), obstruction along the reproductive tract or utilized to perform testicular sperm retrieval.

Egg Donation

Egg donation is an option if you are unable to use your own eggs or the outcome for success of using your eggs is considered extremely poor. During this process, the recipient has been on natural hormones to prepare and synchronize her uterus with the egg donor to ultimately receive the embryo.

Since the 1980s, egg donation had always involved using a young woman to stimulate her ovaries, retrieve her eggs, and then donate her fresh eggs to the recipient. Since 2012, egg freezing has no longer been labelled experimental by ASRM, and women and IVF clinics have increasingly relied upon egg donor banks to supply eggs that are thawed and inseminated to develop embryos as in a fresh cycle.

Fresh vs. frozen donor eggs is a hotly debated topic in reproductive medicine. The current consensus is that frozen eggs may have a slightly lower success rate than fresh eggs. The advantage of frozen eggs is their ease of use and a reduction in cost. Either option results in a much higher chance for a baby rather than using the eggs of a women with severe DOR, particularly in women above age 39 due to a decline in quality.

If you receive an embryo from a donated egg, you should know there may be a higher risk of preeclampsia, a potentially serious pregnancy condition that can cause very high blood pressure and reduce blood flow to the baby, resulting in serious health problems for mom and baby. I advise you to inform your OB/GYN that your pregnancy was from donor eggs so you can be monitored for preeclampsia but also so your baby can have an appropriate risk assessment for chromosomal abnormalities. What does this mean? As you know, as a woman exceeds age 35, her risk of having a baby with Down syndrome (DS) begins to become more of a concern, as well as for all chromosomal abnormalities. A good estimate for the baby's risk of having DS: 1 in 365 pregnancies will have DS for moms at age 35; 1 in 100 pregnancies at age 40. These estimates are based on the woman's age when she conceived. If you used donor eggs, then the risk is based on the age of the donor. This is why your OB/GYN should know you used an egg donor.

The success rate for egg donation is fairly high. The CDC states that over 55 percent of transfers utilizing fresh embryos from donor eggs result in a birth.

Surrogacy

This form of third-party reproduction needs to be clarified because the terms have changed: gestational carrier (GC) is a woman who carries a pregnancy for an intended parent (IP), resulting from an embryo transfer using the IP eggs or donor eggs with IP sperm or donor sperm; a surrogate is a woman who donates her own egg(s) and carries the pregnancy for the IP who used partner or donor sperm, whereby the pregnancy may result from natural conception or IUI as well as IVF. More simply, GC is when there are three different parties involved in the pregnancy (carrier, egg, sperm). A surrogacy simply involves this woman and the sperm source.

Gestational surrogacy is when IVF is used to transfer in a surrogate an embryo of the intended mother's eggs and the father's sperm (or donor gametes of either or both). Live birth rates for IVF with gestational surrogacy, especially using egg donation, are the most successful outcomes in ART because the issues of a uterine factor and egg factor are virtually eliminated, if not dramatically reduced.

In Conclusion

Treatment options for fertility continue to increase. The basic choices when using your eggs and uterus are IUI and IVF. Third-party reproduction—such as egg donation, sperm donation, and/or a gestational carrier—continues to grow in popularity. The correct path for you should be evidence based and include considerations of psychological acceptance and financial commitment.

CHAPTER 18

Embryo Testing and Genetics

The final frontier of any fertility treatment cycle is a live birth—but the penultimate event is embryo implantation. An abnormal embryo based on its chromosomes usually will not implant or it will miscarry. So how do we stack the odds in our favor? Since we can study the embryo, fertility specialists usually focus on improving implantation through IVF. It stands to reason, because IVF has the highest monthly fertility rate of all treatment options. Trying to select the "best" embryo to transfer into your uterus from an IVF cycle has been the Holy Grail of all research in the field of ART.

The most challenging aspect is to determine which embryo is optimal for transfer. In the past, the gold standard method of embryo selection was grading the embryo by appearance, known as morphology. In fact, only approximately 56 percent of embryos will be chromosomally normal if selected by an embryologist in this manner.

What made us start looking at the embryo? Well, the genetic knowledge that more than two-thirds of miscarriages are associated with a chromosomally abnormal embryo is a very compelling statistic which prompted us to study the embryo further. In other words, if we were able to perform an analysis on the embryos in the laboratory prior to transfer, would this improve the pregnancy rate? This question led to PGT.

MOST IMPORTANT FACTORS IN DETERMINING A SUCCESSFUL IVF OUTCOME

1. Endometrium: The lining of the uterus to be receptive while secreting essential proteins for implantation

2. Embryo transfer: The ability for the physician to carefully, without trauma, and accurately transfer the embryo into the optimal location in the upper part of the uterus (fundus)

3. Embryo integrity: The genetic and structural stability of the embryo to develop and communicate with the endometrium for implantation and proceed with normal development

Preimplantation Genetic Testing for Aneuploidy (PGT-A)

PGT-A refers to the technique where embryos from presumed chromosomally normal genetic parents are screened for aneuploidy (the condition where chromosomal regions or numbers are present in extra or fewer copies than normal, typically causing miscarriage). An aneuploid embryo that does not miscarry can result in the birth of a child with special needs due to complex physical and neurologic problems, for example, Down syndrome. PGT-A can screen for this type of scenario and can reduce the miscarriage rate following the transfer of a chromosomally normal embryo.

FAST CHROMOSOME LESSON

- All of us normally have 23 pairs of chromosomes, each containing hundreds to thousands of genes: one set from our mother and the other from our father.
- The 22 pairs are called autosomes; the last pair are sex chromosomes.
- The normal female karyotype (chromosome set) is 46, XX.
- The normal male karyotype is 46, XY.

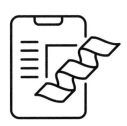

BACKGROUND

Prior to embryo testing on a blastocyst embryo (an embryo that consists of more than 100 cells and grown 5 or 6 days, following egg retrieval, which is the current limit of development in a laboratory and is the stage the embryo naturally enters the uterine cavity), PGT-A was performed on cleavage stage embryos (embryos that have divided to 2 to 4 cells two days after egg retrieval or 6 to 8 cells on day 3 of embryo development), usually on day-three of embryo development. Throughout the 2000s, testing of day-three embryos was thought to significantly improve the implantation rate and live birth rate following embryo transfer. And then, everything changed.

In 2007, a landmark article in the prestigious *New England Journal of Medicine* entitled "In vitro fertilization with preimplantation genetic screening" showed preimplantation genetic screening (PGS as it was then called) did not improve the pregnancy rate. What's worse? PGS *decreased* it! Almost immediately, PGS stopped being performed. (*N Engl J Med.* 2007 Jul 5; 357(1): 9–17)

PGT 2.0

> As women age, the percentage of chromosomally abnormal embryos tested continues to increase—from less than 35 percent under age 30, to more than 60 percent over age 40.

PGT-A offers comprehensive chromosome screening (CCS) to determine the complete karyotype of an embryo. This procedure is performed on day five to six of embryo development at the blastocyst stage. Approximately five to seven cells are delicately removed from the outer part of the embryo called the trophectoderm (future placenta) and then sent to a specialized laboratory for CCS while the embryo is frozen; the testing usually takes up to one week.

Following egg retrieval, embryos are capable of being transferred to the uterus up to day five of development. Once the embryo passes day five of development in a fresh IVF cycle, there is a lack of synchrony with the lining of the uterus (endometrium) as well as an inability to maintain the growing embryo in the laboratory culture.

Rarely is the genetic laboratory performing the analysis at the same location as the IVF center, so most programs offer the patient a two-step process: The embryos are immediately frozen following biopsy and then once the genetic information is returned, the patient undergoes a FET cycle the following month.

Fortunately, due to advances in freezing using a process called vitrification, FET cycles allow for similar pregnancy rates as fresh cycles. If one focuses only on CCS cycles, then FET cycles may result in a higher pregnancy rate.

Why do patients choose PGT-A?

- Unexplained recurrent miscarriage (RM)
- Women over 37 years of age to improve embryo selection
- Desiring family balancing (by selecting the gender of the offspring)

While PGT-A has been used in patients with RM, there is no definitive evidence for an improved outcome. However, due to its potential for shortening the time to pregnancy, PGT-A may be of increased value for women of advanced reproductive age. This technology can also reduce the risk of multiple gestations through the enhanced selection of a single normal embryo for transfer.

Increasingly, many of you are asking about family balancing by selecting the gender of the baby. While IVF with chromosome testing is considered the gold standard, sperm sorting with IUI is a much less expensive option. This sorting is based on the molecular weight of the X- and Y- bearing sperm, with X being heavier. The outcomes with a pregnancy are about 80 to 90 percent for the preferred gender. IVF with PGT-A has a less than 1 percent error rate but is much more expensive. To maximize your chance for gender selection with IVF, you can add sperm sorting prior to insemination of your eggs.

PGT-A FOR ALL?

The field of IVF continues to evolve rapidly. Patients are justifiably anxious for improved outcomes and physicians are understandably pressured to accommodate them. However, this should not supersede the safe implementation of technology. I have two major concerns over the universal application of PGT-A:

1. The chromosomal content of the embryo is not the only determining factor for successful implantation. Miscarriages can occur following transfer of embryos with normal chromosomes. The rate reported in medical studies is typically less than 10 percent, but not all studies have shown a lower pregnancy loss rate compared to not using PGT-A. While chromosomes are very important for a successful healthy pregnancy, they are not an assurance of the outcome.

2. The information gained from PGT-A can uncover a phenomenon called mosaicism. Sometimes the PGT-A report will give us the result of one of more mosaic embryos. This means the embryo has two genetically different sets of cell lines—one normal and one abnormal, as opposed to one cell line.

Now there is the question of how to proceed with mosaic embryos. Does this consequence dismiss the use of these embryos? Or is it indeterminate enough to avoid an embryo transfer?

Some researchers decided to take the chance and transfer mosaic embryos. The patients were apparently well informed of the risks of the unknown outcome. The results? Mosaic embryos transferred resulted in a lower live birth rates, higher miscarriage rate, but no higher risk of birth defects seen in the children born compared to normal embryos that were transferred.

So, here are my thoughts. There is too much enthusiasm for advances in IVF without enough oversight and assurance of safety. By asking patients who are desperate for a baby to provide consent for a new but incompletely understood procedure with unknown long-term effects, physicians can potentially exploit a patient's desperation. Currently it is premature to recommend PGT-A to all patients—given the lack of definitive improvement in time to pregnancy, risk of embryo damage, and cost of testing, along with the need for a frozen embryo replacement cycle (since the fresh embryo transfer is deferred due to embryo testing). There is evidence to support the use PGT-A in women who are 38 years of age and older to improve the chance for a live birth following an embryo transfer.

In addition to PGT-A, two other methods for determining the optimal embryo to improve pregnancy rates, while reducing the number of embryos transferred and reducing multiple gestation, are time-lapse photography and metabolomics.

Time-lapse Photography

This technology (repetitive photographs of the embryos every five minutes while they are in the incubator) has been shown to increase the ability to predict which embryos will develop to the blastocyst stage but has not yet been determined to predict live birth rates.

Bottom Line: Despite excitement over another tool, time-lapse photography has not been shown to improve outcome with IVF.

Metabolomics

By analyzing culture media surrounding the embryos, metabolic by-products secreted into that media solution are tested using biomarkers to assess embryo viability. This is very new technology and, obviously, does not involve disturbing the embryo. We anxiously await more information!

What About Testing for Inherited Genetic Diseases?

Preimplantation genetic testing for monogenic disorders (PGT-M) refers to the embryo analysis when one or both parents are carriers for the same single-gene defect (mutation), and testing is performed to determine if the embryo has received the mutation from one or both parents that will result in a serious disease. PGT-M enables people with an inheritable condition to avoid passing that condition on to their children, screen for cancer-related gene mutations, or select an embryo who would be a suitable donor to provide cord blood or stem cells for transplantation to a sibling with a fatal illness.

Developed in the United Kingdom in the mid-1980s, PGT-M initially focused on determining gender as an indirect means of avoiding an X-linked recessive disorders. Remember: The sex chromosomes are XX for a female and XY for a male. X-linked recessive disorders affect a child when only one X exists, which means only boys will be afflicted with X-linked recessive diseases.

In 1989 in London, the first unaffected child was born following PGT-M performed for an X-linked disorder. Since then the indications for PGT-M have become well established, and it is currently available for most known genetic mutations (such as cystic fibrosis, sickle cell anemia, Tay-Sachs disease, hemophilias, and muscular dystrophy).

PGT-M tests the embryos in the same manner as PGT-A at the blastocyst stage.

CRISPR—The Game Changer

While PGT-A and PGT-M are still evolving aspects of reproductive genetics, the next big thing in reproductive genetics could be CRISPR, which many are saying will herald the beginning of a golden age in genetic engineering.

CRISPR, which stands for "clustered regularly interspaced short palindromic repeats," has allowed researchers to slice the genome in human cells at sites of their choosing. In other words, it's selective gene editing and it works as follows: Scientists design and synthesize a piece of RNA, one of the kinds of genetic material in all human cells, that matches a specific sequence of DNA. This piece of RNA is called a Guide RNA and the DNA sequence it matches is called the Target DNA. The Guide RNA then carries special molecules to the Target DNA and the molecules cut the two DNA strands within the target—much as film for a movie used to be cut as it was being edited. Next, where the Target DNA was cut, a "repair template" introduces a new genetic sequence to the DNA, guiding it to do "good" things for the body instead of the "bad" things that were cut out.

Until recently, editing individual genes—whether the cells were plant, mouse, or human—was a slow and often futile process. But now, with CRISPR, we have an effective and efficient ability to snip individual genes or even insert new ones in their place. CRISPR's monumental advances in gene-editing have made it possible to tweak the DNA of different organisms with incredible, unprecedented precision.

So far, some of the most promising applications for CRISPR include Alzheimer's and cancer treatments. Yet, while CRISPR could include gene editing in human embryos for coveted traits like high intelligence or muscular stature, most scientists say this potential use is much more scientifically challenging and less important than other applications. With 3 billion base pairs, the human genome is so massive that complex modifications will be a major hurdle even with CRISPR. Plus, embryo editing is ethically fraught, and it will likely be many more years before any scientist in the United States gets approval to try it (although China and other countries may move faster).

We also need to remember that any such edits/changes to an embryo's genomes would almost certainly be passed down to subsequent generations, breaching an ethical line that has typically been a line not to be crossed.

In Conclusion

Whether you undergo natural attempts at conception, fertility medications with IUI, or IVF, the field of reproductive medicine still cannot explain why a normal embryo does not implant or it miscarries.

We are in an amazing era of technological advances in IVF. However, as physicians, we must remember to remain ethical and have integrity, namely, the fact something can be performed does not necessarily mean it should and certainly only after intense oversight to ensure safety and proven outcomes.

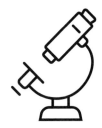

CHAPTER 19

Financing Infertility Treatments

First, a note: Not all the financial options discussed in this chapter have been vetted personally by me and I cannot endorse the ones I have not vetted. Please research your best options with your providers and your insurance carriers.

Infertility is a physical, emotional, and financial investment with all three factors being equivalent in their impact. In states where infertility insurance is mandated, the fertility specialist focuses most of the consultation on treatment options and leaves the financial arrangements to the insurance counselor of the practice. Alternatively, in states that do not have mandated infertility insurance, a large portion of the consult with your physician is spent on the cost of each medical treatment option. While this is certainly appropriate and vital to offer cost-effective treatment options, extensive financial conversations add unnecessary stress to the already stressed infertility patient/couple. The goal of this chapter is to provide you with more understanding and resources for financing your fertility, typically IVF treatment.

The following programs will not cover 100 percent of your infertility treatment costs; however, some in combination may cover a large portion of it. People who successfully raise funds for IVF despite financial hardship usually do so by combining several different offers and then financing the rest. Because not all these offers can be used in tandem, you may need to run the numbers for a variety of different program combinations and see which is best for your unique situation.

In addition, you should begin taking steps to improve your credit rating as soon as possible, as many of the best financing options require good or excellent credit. No one will deny that IVF is expensive. These financing options, especially when combined, can make IVF financially possible for many people who struggle to conceive.

IVF Financing Option 1: Health Insurance

Many people assume that their regular health insurance will not cover IVF, but this is not always true. There are currently 17 states that require some form of coverage for fertility treatments by standard health insurance plans, although the amount of coverage varies by state and by the insurance plan; 11 states require IVF coverage and 7 states require fertility preservation for cancer patients and others at risk of medically-induced infertility.

Even if your state does not mandate IVF coverage, your plan may still cover some of the costs.

The first step to financing your IVF is to find out whether your state mandates coverage, whether your plan offers it, and what expenses will be left afterward.

Insurance coverage is one of your first-line IVF financing options.

IVF Financing Option 2: Loans Against Assets

A couple TTC often owns assets besides cash in checking and savings accounts. For example, many people have equity in a home, a life insurance policy, or a retirement investment account such as a 401k. You do not have to liquidate these assets to use them to fund IVF; in many cases, you can take out a personal loan using these and other assets as collateral. For example, many people take out a home equity loan to help with IVF financing and other fertility treatments.

Financing Option 3: Fertility Grants

There are several charitable foundations, such as the Cade Foundation and B.U.M.P.S., that give out cash grants to people who need but cannot afford fertility treatments. These grants are not enough money to cover the full cost, but they can take a large chunk out of your bill and be combined with other assistance and financing programs if you can show financial need.

A list of resources for infertility treatment grants can be found at the RESOLVE website, resolve.org.

Option 4: Help from Family and Friends

While it can be embarrassing to fundraise among your loved ones, they likely want to help you. Even smaller gifts can add up immensely. This gives your loved ones a chance to give you the gift of a lifetime: a family.

Consider having a fundraiser or signing up with Deposit a Gift or Go Fund Me to help fund your IVF treatments. This online cash gift registry allows friends and family to contribute to your IVF fund, which collectively can come to a substantial amount of money. The cash is then sent to you in a check or direct deposited into your bank account in a simple, streamlined process. (Contact: www.depositagift.com or www.gofundme.com)

Option 5: The Assisted Reproduction Insurance Program

This program through New Life Agency Inc. offers insurance plans that cover fertility services, including IVF. In addition, partial refunds are given if pregnancy is not achieved. This plan requires that you see a doctor who is part of the preferred provider network, but you can ask your doctor to join if they are not listed. There are also discounts on common fertility prescriptions when bought at Walgreens Pharmacy.

As with any health insurance policy, it is important to read the fine print and understand exactly what services and treatments will be covered. (Contact: www. newlifeagency.com)

IVF Financing Option 6: The ARC Fertility Program

This program was founded by reproductive endocrinologists in 1997 and is run by Advanced Reproductive Care, Inc (ARC). I endorse the use of this program. The ARC Fertility Program offers a national list of physicians and clinics that will accept less expensive package pricing for up to three live IVF cycles and three frozen cycles. There is also package pricing available for other common fertility treatments, such as IUI. There are a few downsides to this financing option. Full payment for the package must be made in advance to Advanced Reproductive Care, who will forward it to your doctor. In addition, no refunds are given if you conceive the first cycle and do not use the others in your package. In order to qualify for this program, you must fill out applications for both the fertility treatments and the pharmaceuticals.

The applications can both be found online at www.arcfertility.com.

Option 7: The Assure IVF Refund Program

Like the ARC program, the Assure IVF Refund program allows people to pay a lower fixed fee for three live and three frozen cycles. I also endorse this program. However, it also has the benefit of a refund program. If the patient does not have a successful conception, pregnancy, and birth, they get 80 to 100 percent of their money back. Rather than paying upfront as with the ARC program, Assure IVF Refund Program offers financing through American Healthcare Lending. This makes their services more accessible to many couples. In order to get this flat fee, patients must fill out an application and meet eligibility requirements. This program may not be available in all states. (Contact: www.assureivf.com)

Option 8: Compassionate Care

This is a pharmaceutical-assistance program run by EMD Serono, one of the leading manufacturers of fertility medications. I endorse the use of this program. Patients who can show financial need can get a percent discount or $10 off each prescription. Eligibility for this program is determined by gross household income and other factors. The details and application can be found at the company website. In addition, veterans who do not qualify for the veteran-specific Compassionate Corps program can get 25 percent off their fertility medications even if they do not qualify for the 50 to 75 percent discount. (Contact: www.emdseronofertility.com)

Option 9: Compassionate Corps

This is another pharmaceutical-discount program offered by fertility drug maker EMD Serono, and one I also endorse. This program offers free fertility medications for retired veterans who are infertile due to an injury acquired while in active military service or their spouses. In addition to being infertile due to an injury occurring while serving in the military, couples also must not have insurance that covers IVF and must be diagnosed as requiring this procedure by a physician.

The programs offered by EMD Serono can be combined as eligible to cover a great deal of the medications needed for IVF, making this one of the best IVF financing options. (Contact: www.emdseronofertility.com)

IVF Financing Option 10: WINFertility

Another program I endorse is WINFertility, a discounted bundled fee for services rendered at one of its participating clinics. In addition to covering services, this package deal includes medications and other expenses. There are over 100 clinics currently participating in this program. The savings add up to around 40 percent of the cost of getting the same services without a package at retail price.

Treatment packages cover all the expenses for a single round of IVF. There are also bundles for IUI, IVF Freeze and Thaw, and other common fertility treatments.

People who choose to use the WINfertility package at a participating provider can also apply for low interest financing. In addition, there are several side benefits to this infertility financing option. A hotline is available where patients can speak to a trained fertility nurse at any time via a hotline. In addition, there are no restrictions for age or medical condition. (Contact: www.winfertility.com)

Option 11: WINFertilityRx

WINfertilityRX is the other component of WINfertility's bundle option for IVF. I endorse this program as well. The program offers up to 40 percent off fertility medications for people who are paying for them out-of-pocket. In addition, participants get the same access to a trained fertility nurse hotline as people who purchase the treatment package. There are no coupons, forms, cards, or unusual criteria in order to qualify for this program. Patients receive their medications in the mail with free express shipping in the United States, along with a Fertility Order Review that explains how to store and to use the medications in each order. Medications usually arrive one business day after the order is placed. (Contact: www.winfertilityrx.com)

Option 12: Fertility and Reproductive Financing Program

Prosper Healthcare Lending (formerly American Healthcare Lending), which I also endorse, is one of the leading lending agencies for Americans who cannot cover the costs of needed or wanted health treatments. This company's fertility financing options will cover any fertility costs up to $100,000, with up to 84 months to repay the loan and no penalties for people who pay off the loan early. People who wish to get on this loan program must apply online and meet basic financing criteria including a certain credit score and annual income requirements. The application can be completed from any device. An immediate decision is available for loans of less than $35,000. In addition, patients must get their IVF services from an AHCL Fertility and Reproductive Program approved clinic or fertility specialist. (Contact: www.prosperhealthcare.com)

Option 13: Shared Risk 100% Refund Program

This program offers a bundle with six fresh cycles of IVF as well as frozen or donor embryo transfers for one flat fee. If the patient does not have a successful pregnancy and birth, there is a 100 percent refund. In order to be approved, patients must have a complete medical screening and be deemed good candidates for IVF. In addition, women must be less than 39 years old when the last cycle of IVF is completed unless they are using donor eggs. Financing for the Shared Risk 100% Refund Program is offered from Shady Grove Fertility. (Contact: www.shadygrovefertility.com)

Option 14: ReUnite Rx

This program offers fertility financing options for qualifying patients by allowing patients to apply for need-based assistance. Active or veteran military members automatically qualify for a ReUnite Assist 25% discount. ReUnite Oncofertility offers discounted medications for cancer patients who undergo fertility preservation. Discounts are determined based on clinical considerations and financial need. (Contact: www.reuniterx.com)

Option 15: Financing from New Life Agency in Partnership with LightStream

These two companies have collaborated to offer IVF financing options for all kinds of assisted reproduction, including fertility medications, IVF, and surrogacy. Qualifying medications must be purchased from a Walgreens Pharmacy. In order to qualify, patients must have at least good or excellent credit. The loan is processed by LightStream in a paperless online process, with most applicants receiving an almost immediate response. All fertility and assisted reproductive options are covered. If approved, the requested funding will be deposited into the patient's bank account, usually on the same day as application, with no down payment or fees. Financing from New Life Agency in partnership with LightStream is available up to $100,000 with fixed annual interest rates starting at 5.99 percent. No collateral, liens, or other security is necessary, although the required credit rating may be a challenge. (Contact: www. newlifeagency.com)

Financing Option 16: Ferring Reproductive Health

This pharmaceutical savings program covers fertility medications made by Ferring Pharmaceuticals. This program helps patients who do not have insurance covering their pharmaceutical costs. The covered drugs for this program include Endometrin, which allows you to save up to $30 every two weeks with a patient savings card. Up to 50 percent of the cash cost of these drugs is covered. Unlike other pharmaceutical programs, IVF Greenlight has no income requirements or financial documents to submit. All a patient needs in order to get on this discount program is a prescription for a minimum amount of the medications. For example, people only qualify if they have been prescribed ten or more vials of Bravelle or Menopur. For cancer patients interested in preserving their fertility, Ferring Pharmaceuticals and Walgreens have developed the Heart Beat Program. Select fertility medications are at no cost and there are no financial requirements. They also offer select fertility products through Hearts for Heroes for veterans requiring assisted reproduction due to a service-related injury that resulted in infertility. (Contact: www.ferringfertility.com)

Option 17: First Steps Program

This is another pharmaceutical assistance-program, this one offered by DesignRx. I endorse this program. This company is the maker of drugs such as follitropin injectable Follstim, injectable Ganirelix, and Pregynl. Patients who apply for this program should be able to demonstrate hardship, including meeting financial requirements. However, everyone who applies receives some kind of discount, so everyone should apply. Patients need to have a valid prescription for one of the covered drugs at a pharmacy that is in DesignRX's network. DesignRX will issue people who qualify with a card that gives them up to 75 percent off their out-of-pocket cost. This offer cannot be combined with any other offers, such as rebates, free trials, or coupons. However, the discount card can be used repeatedly throughout the year, with participants reapplying every calendar year. (Contact: www.fertilitybydesign.com)

Financing Option 18: Multi-Cycle Discount Plans by Attain Fertility™ Centers

Like many of the programs listed here, Attain Fertility offers a bundle of IVF services for a single low price. This is a program I endorse. There are several different program options, all of which must be received at a fertility clinic that is within the Attain Fertility Centers network.

There are two main programs offered from Attain Fertility: Attain Multi-Cycle Discount Program and Attain Multi-Cycle Discount Program + REFUND. The Attain Multi-Cycle Discount Program offers six IVF cycles total, three fresh cycles, and three FETs. The Attain Multi-Cycle Discount Program + REFUND offers the same number of cycles as the Attain Multi-Cycle Discount Program except that there is a refund if treatment does not result in a successful pregnancy. The refund is 70 percent for patients who are using their own harvested eggs and up to 100 percent for cycles using donor eggs. This is one of the most successful of the package deal programs. Three-quarters of participants had a baby using Attain and only one quarter request a refund.

There are medical requirements to get this program, but they are not stringent. More than 75 percent of applicants are accepted into one of the two programs. There are also donor egg programs for people who likely will not be able to conceive using their own eggs. (Contact: www.attainfertility.com)

Option 20: The IVF Financial Share Program

This is another package deal and refund program, with a few details that set it apart. The first distinction is that treatment must be received at an In Vitro Sciences Center of Excellence, which are available throughout the nation. If the patient is accepted to this program, they will receive a discounted flat fee for up to three fresh and three frozen IVF cycles. If patients do not have a successful conception and pregnancy, they will receive up to a 70 percent discount.

There are a few requirements to qualify for this program; patients must be under the age of 38 unless they are using donor eggs. They need to apply and submit detailed medical records showing they are a good candidate for IVF. People who choose this infertility payment option will need to either pay in advance for their treatment package or qualify for financing through Springstone Patient Financing. (Contact: www.invitrosciences.com)

In Conclusion

The disease of infertility carries an emotional and physical challenge to all of you. The additional financial burden, which often can be a deal-breaker toward proceeding with a desired management plan, is more than you all should have to endure. You should be your best advocate by carefully reviewing your insurance benefits package with your human resources department to help you navigate the financial challenges along your journey.

The resources outlined in this chapter will hopefully be a useful guide to you and reduce your burden, at least to some degree.

CHAPTER 20

Early Pregnancy Complications

All pregnancies require careful monitoring in the first trimester to ensure the implanted embryo is developing normally and in the appropriate location. Infertility patients may be at a higher risk of pregnancy loss—depending upon their treatment to conceive and their medical history. A pregnancy that miscarries may have initially developed inside the uterine cavity (called an IUP), outside the uterine cavity (called an ectopic pregnancy), or at an unknown location (called a PUL).

How do we know if your pregnancy is healthy in the first trimester? These are the top six factors for avoiding complications during the beginning of your pregnancy.

1. hCG Levels

The blood levels and rate of rise of hCG can either be reassuring or be a red flag that indicates more testing is needed. Blood levels for this pregnancy hormone, in the early stages of pregnancy, normally rise at a minimum of 49 percent in 48 hours. While a low percentage of normal pregnancies may demonstrate an initial abnormal rate of hCG rise, the contrary can also occur—for example, when a low percentage of abnormal or ectopic pregnancies may show an initial normal rate of hCG rise.

By the time your hCG level is above 3500 IU/L, an IUP should be seen by TUVS. If no pregnancy is seen, or at the very least a gestational sac, then we have a high concern for an ectopic pregnancy.

Your risk for an ectopic pregnancy resulting from a natural conception is 1 to 2 percent but increases from an IVF cycle to approximately 5 percent and up to 10 percent with a history of a tubal surgery or a prior ectopic pregnancy. Following a frozen embryo replacement cycle, the risk for an ectopic pregnancy is 65 percent lower than following a fresh embryo transfer. Rare but real, the incidence of a heterotopic pregnancy (a simultaneous pregnancy of an intrauterine and ectopic) is 1 in 10,000 natural conceptions, but dramatically increases to 1 percent of pregnancies occurring as a result of IVF.

The risk factors for ectopic pregnancy are

- Prior ectopic pregnancy
- History of tubal surgery, including a bilateral tubal ligation
- History of STIs
- Currently using an intrauterine device (IUD)
- Pregnancy as a result of IVF, particularly a fresh embryo transfer
- Tobacco use
- DES exposure (a drug potentially taken by your mother while she was pregnant with you)

Traditional treatment for an ectopic pregnancy has been by surgery to remove the affected tube via opening the woman's abdomen. Advances in laparoscopy have reduced the invasiveness of tubal surgery to a same-day outpatient procedure. Depending on the degree of damage to the affected tube, the surgeon may be able to avoid removing the tube by simply opening the tube and removing the pregnancy. However, this method can result in left-behind pregnancy tissue called a persistent ectopic pregnancy in up to 20 percent of surgeries that may require medical treatment with methotrexate therapy.

The outcome for future fertility after an ectopic pregnancy depends on the condition of the nonaffected fallopian tube. When that tube is normal, subsequent ongoing pregnancy rates are the same (approximately 60 to 70 percent) whether the treatment was tubal removing (salpingectomy) or tubal sparing (salpingostomy).

Since the early 1990s, a cancer chemotherapy drug (methotrexate or MTX) has been used to treat a woman with ectopic pregnancy diagnosed in the early stages. Methotrexate has an effectiveness of approximately 85 percent, when prescribed at levels of hCG less than 10,000 IU/L, and 95 percent at levels less than 5000 IU/L. Treatment with methotrexate does come with its risks, though, including increased abdominal girth, an increase in hCG, vaginal spotting or bleeding, and abdominal pain. The drug itself can cause gastric distress, dizziness, and in rare cases, sever neutropenia, reversible alopecia, and pneumonitis.

2. Thyroid

During the first trimester of pregnancy, the baby cannot produce adequate thyroid hormone until 10 to 13 weeks of pregnancy, so it relies on mom's thyroid hormone. Without adequate thyroid for mom and baby, higher risks for pregnancy loss, baby development, and health problems during and after the pregnancy can occur.

HYPOTHYROID-RELATED NEGATIVE IMPACT ON MOM AND BABY IF LEFT UNTREATED		
	MOM	**BABY**
PREGNANCY	Anemia, heart disease, elevated blood pressure; higher C-section rate	Growth restriction; increased mortality
DELIVERY	Higher C-section rate	Higher miscarriage rate
LONG TERM	Postpartum depression and high blood pressure; breast feeding problems	Impaired neurologic and intellectual development

Some background for understanding thyroid: you can have an overactive thyroid (hyperthyroidism) or underactive thyroid (hypothyroidism). Both conditions, if left improperly treated, can cause significant health and pregnancy problems, including infertility. There are preconditions to both diseases, subclinical hyperthyroidism and hypothyroidism, which means the labs show a mild abnormality but you have little to no symptoms. One last condition is the presence of antibodies to your thyroid, specifically TPO, which are often associated with thyroid disease but may be present before the disease is diagnosed. The presence of TPO has been shown to increase miscarriage and reduce live birth rates (from a study of the National Institutes of Health).

In pregnant women with true hypothyroidism (when the body lacks enough thyroid hormone), the Endocrine Society recommends TSH levels of less than 2.5 mIU/L during pregnancy because elevations beyond this dosage increase negative obstetrical outcomes.

There is no consensus on treating TSH levels in patients with levels above 2.5 mIU/L and still in the normal range or with subclinical hypothyroidism. The pendulum has really swung when we look at the issue of who would benefit from thyroid hormone during pregnancy (outside of those with true hypothyroidism). Let's be clear—there is no evidence of impaired outcome in baby with mom's TSH levels between 2.5 and 4 mIU/L during prepregnancy. The only situations that appear to impair reproductive outcome, namely, miscarriage and preterm birth, are the presence of thyroid antibodies (TPO) and subclinical hypothyroidism (TSH levels above the upper limit of normal, but a normal level of circulating thyroid hormone). In these two conditions, low dose thyroid hormone replacement appears to be of value.

Bottom Line: You should have your thyroid checked if you have infertility and need thyroid hormone replacement, to keep TSH < 2.5 mIU/L, when you have thyroid disease (true or subclinical) or thyroid antibodies.

3. Bleeding

Is there anything more frightening than vaginal bleeding during pregnancy, especially to a woman who has tried for years to conceive? Well it happens in 15 to 25 percent of pregnant women in the first trimester. Any bleeding causes alarm, but only heavy bleeding is more likely associated with miscarriage, which can occur 25 to 50 percent of the time.

Until the location of your pregnancy has been confirmed, hopefully inside your uterus rather than an ectopic, you need to notify your obstetrician if you have vaginal bleeding. The evaluation of vaginal bleeding in pregnancy consists of your doctor performing a pelvic examination, obtaining hCG blood levels (as reviewed above), and a vaginal ultrasound to determine the location and health of the pregnancy. If the pregnancy is intrauterine but bleeding continues, then close monitoring throughout the first trimester is necessary. To manage vaginal bleeding, there is no good medical evidence to having your blood progesterone measured, using natural vaginal progesterone, or bedrest. We recommend avoiding sexual intercourse while bleeding to reduce the low risk of infection.

Of importance, a RhoGAM injection (used to prevent a complication of pregnancy known as Rhesus disease, or hemolytic disease, of the newborn) is necessary within three days of bleeding onset in those of you who are Rh factor negative and your partner is Rh factor positive or unknown. This injection reduces the risk of you developing antibodies against the red blood cells of the fetus that can cause problems ranging from mild anemia up to fetal death.

4. Fetal Heart Rate (FHR)

Thanks to the use of Doppler technology, you can hear your fetus' heartbeat as early as six weeks into your pregnancy (we use the term embryo until eight weeks of pregnancy). The normal FHR ranges between 120 and 160. In the first trimester, a repeatedly below normal FHR (especially when associated with poor fetal growth) is very concerning for a healthy pregnancy outcome. However, a single FHR below normal reading, especially less than seven weeks of pregnancy, should not diagnose an abnormal fetus because early stage of development and physiologic changes can result in FHR fluctuations.

Once an FHR is heard, the risk of miscarriage is reduced—the rate of loss after ultrasound demonstrates fetal cardiac motion at an EGA of > 8 weeks is less than 5 percent—but higher in patients with recurrent miscarriage (up to 20 percent).

5. Fetal Measurement

With accurate dating of conception using a women's menstrual cycle or, more optimally, by an OPK, a vaginal ultrasound can measure the fetus to determine whether growth is consistent with the fetus's EGA.

As with FHR, one measurement does not usually make a diagnosis of an abnormal pregnancy due to the range of error using ultrasound technology and the inaccuracies of the definite conception date with a spontaneous pregnancy. However, recent guidelines define a nonviable pregnancy as an embryo measuring greater than 7 millimeters (0.3 inches) without a heart rate.

Infertility patients who have undergone ART (i.e., IVF) have a much more precise conception date. The earlier the ultrasound is obtained during the pregnancy, the more accurate the measurement. This means that if the embryo/fetus is measuring smaller at an earlier stage in pregnancy and the conception date is accurate, the health of the pregnancy is worrisome.

6. Multiple Pregnancy

When a woman is TTC but can't, nothing seems to spark the sharp pain of that experience more than the sight of two little babies, one swaddled in pink and the other in blue, nestled in a double stroller. "Two for the price of one," she might think. "Why shouldn't I do IVF once, conceive twins or triplets, get it over with, and live happily ever after?"

According to the SART, the objective of infertility treatment should be the birth of a single, healthy child—with "single" being the operative word. A multiple gestation (meaning twins or greater) can pose serious health concerns for mother and babies, as well as a financial burden for the parents and society.

Contrary to popular belief, non-IVF fertility treatment (i.e., ovulation induction and ovarian stimulation) is responsible for a much higher percentage of multiple births than IVF fertility treatment. From 1998 to 2011, the percentage of IVF twins increased from 10 to 17 percent, while the incidence of triplet and higher-order births decreased by 29 percent (due to SART recommending reducing the number of embryos transferred).

The disparity between the outcomes of IVF versus non-IVF fertility treatment stems from the lack of control over the number of eggs exposed to sperm in the fallopian tube, as well as the number of embryos reaching the uterus. In other words, IVF allows for a decision on the number of embryos entering the uterine cavity, while non-IVF fertility treatment does not.

The result is that the rate of twins from IVF procedures has remained relatively stable, while the rate of triplets (or more) from IVF has undergone a dramatic decline. This reduction in triplets or higher births from IVF is due to the concerted effort of SART and clinics to reduce the number of embryos transferred.

MATERNAL COMPLICATIONS IN MULTIPLE PREGNANCIES

The most common complications of multiple gestation pregnancies (along with their risk based on number of fetuses) are preeclampsia, gestational diabetes, preterm labor, and early delivery. Other risks of multiple gestation include excess weight gain, anemia, worsening of pregnancy-associated gastrointestinal symptoms, back pain, shortness of breath, umbilical hernias, severe nausea, and vomiting.

PREECLAMPSIA

This is a dangerous (although rarely fatal) condition in which the pregnant woman's blood pressure becomes elevated in conjunction with large amounts of protein excreted in the urine. In severe cases, delivery of the fetus(es) must be performed irrespective of gestational age to avoid serious harm, including death, to the mother. A valuable resource is the American College of Obstetricians and Gynecologists (ACOG) website at www.acog.org which provides several important links on preeclampsia.

GESTATIONAL DIABETES

Women pregnant with twins or higher number multiples are twice or even more likely to experience gestational diabetes (a type of diabetes that is first seen in a pregnant woman who did not have diabetes before she was pregnant). Serious complications are rare and include preterm delivery and a baby whose size is large for its gestational age.

MORBIDITY AND MORTALITY IN MULTIPLE PREGNANCIES

Multiple gestation tends to significantly increase the risks to babies in several important categories. While survival for most premature newborns at 23 weeks has increased from zero to about 65 percent over the last 20 years, each week the fetus remains inside the mom significantly increases survival, based on birth weight, to 90 percent by 27 to 28 weeks of gestational age, and by about 95 percent by 33 weeks of gestational age. Nevertheless, complications from preterm birth do occur and include the following: chronic lung disease, developmental delay, and growth reduction, hearing impairment, intraventricular hemorrhage, respiratory distress syndrome, and others.

COMPLICATIONS FOR THE FAMILY FROM A MULTIPLE PREGNANCY

1. Financial strain—This is especially true if one or more of the babies have special medical or developmental needs.

2. Logistical strain—This pertains to matters such as managing work and childcare, transportation, routine household tasks, and breastfeeding.

3. Emotional strain—Emotional challenges can be made worse if the mother experiences long-term postpartum depression.

WHY RISK A MULTIPLE GESTATION?

One of the rationales behind transferring more than one embryo into your uterus is your worry that you may only be able to afford one IVF cycle. So you opt to "put all your eggs in one basket" and may encourage your physician to be more aggressive.

However, please note that "aggressive" and "proactive" are not equivalent terms in this situation. As an alternative, what if you decided to limit the number of embryos you wish your physician to transfer? If twins or triplets are born prematurely with health complications, the resultant financial cost can quickly become burdensome.

Fortunately, there is very good news about this alternative. More studies show that elective single fresh embryo transfer (then one frozen embryo, if needed) has a similar overall live birth rate and much lower risk of multiple birth compared with transferring two fresh embryos. Furthermore, transferring a single chromosomally normal embryo using preimplantation genetic screening has an equivalent live birth rate compared to transferring two untested embryos.

GUIDELINES YOU CAN LIVE BY

The ASRM and the SART have copublished guidelines on the number of embryos that should be transferred during an IVF cycle for women. These guidelines are based on PGT, the woman's age, and day of embryo development; a favorable prognosis is usually a prior success with IVF and if there are extra embryos frozen. For example, embryos on day 3 (cleavage stage) of development stage have a lower chance of success, per embryo, than day 5 embryos (blastocysts). To summarize, women younger than age 38 should receive a single embryo—cleavage stage or blastocyst—if their prognosis is favorable as outlined previously. Women of any age should receive a single embryo if the PGT results are normal. As a woman ages, the number of embryos she has to transfer declines.

It is important to note the guidelines apply to IVF cycles where you are using your own eggs. And, if you are undergoing egg donor IVF cycles, these guidelines apply to the age of the egg donor, not the age of the recipient.

While exceptions to the ASRM/SART guidelines are allowed, any exceptions should be limited and only considered under unique medical circumstances. You should discuss your specific situation with your infertility specialist and embryologist and determine if the guidelines are applicable in your case.

In Conclusion

While these complications can certainly be scary to consider, there are ways you can reduce your risks:

- Ectopic pregnancy or bleeding—Until you confirm the location of your pregnancy, you should promptly notify your OB/GYN of bleeding or abdominal pain. If you are Rh− and your partner's blood type is Rh+ or unknown, you should receive RhoGam (see page 162).
- Thyroid—Treat with thyroid hormone if you have positive TPO antibodies or true or subclinical thyroid disease. Pregnancy will increase your thyroid hormone requirement so your dose may need to be adjusted.
- Multiple births—When possible, proceed with elective single embryo transfer according to the guidelines on page 164.

We spend the most time on the risk of multiple births because this has the highest percentage chance to occur (if you transfer more than one embryo) than the other ones. Will all multiple births result in a poor outcome? Thankfully no, but the decision will have long-lasting implications. The best solution may be a frank discussion with your infertility specialist.

When you are proactive, knowledgeable, and in control, you can proceed with cautious optimism, while building toward, and then creating, the family of your dreams.

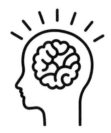

CHAPTER 21

Preserving Fertility from Cancer

The field of *oncofertility* focuses on the importance of maintaining fertility in cancer patients using a multidisciplinary approach that includes the fields of oncology, reproductive endocrinology, and molecular biology.

Owing to the increasing success of oncologists over the past four decades, patients diagnosed with cancer are surviving longer, and their care now focuses on improving quality of life and long-term health. Chemotherapy and radiation, the standards of care in cancer treatment, result in significant gonadotoxicity (toxic to the female gonad or ovary and male gonad or testis), impairing a woman's (and man's) fertility. As a result, cancer patients in their reproductive years are faced with another life crisis—preserving their fertility.

Over 100,000 women 45 years of age and younger are diagnosed with cancer each year.

Between 1990 and 2008, overall cancer death rates decreased by 23 percent in men and 15 percent in women—representing approximately one million lives saved. Approximately 77 percent of cancer patients diagnosed younger than 45 years of age survive longer than five years. These rates are continuing to improve for the four most serious cancers: lung, colon, breast, and prostate.

Consequently, in 2006, the American Society of Clinical Oncology recommended, "As part of the consent prior to therapy, oncologists should address the possibility of infertility with patients as early in treatment planning as possible," and "Fertility preservation is an important, if not necessary, consideration when planning cancer treatment in reproductive-age patients."

Not all oncologists will address fertility preservation: 82 to 84 percent of medical and radiation oncologists and 51 percent of surgical oncologists "always/often" discuss fertility preservation with their patients; and 24 to 31 percent of all oncologists "rarely/never" refer for fertility preservation.

Fertility preservation options depend on many factors. Your age will provide insight to your ovarian reserve to contemplate the utility of fertility preservation. The tumor type, stage, and treatment plan determine the time available, if any, to proceed with an emergency IVF cycle. Your relationship status may influence the choice of freezing eggs or embryos because IVF requires insemination with sperm unless egg freezing is chosen. Lastly, and most importantly, the psychological impact on you should always be addressed.

Based on the stage and aggressiveness of your cancer, your health may preclude or allow an IVF cycle. Insurance coverage for IVF will determine the cost of fertility preservation treatment to the patient. Only a handful of states in the United States mandate insurance coverage for fertility preservation in cancer patients but there is a strong movement to increase coverage nationwide.

For many years, postpubertal males who are being treated for cancer have preserved their fertility by cryopreserving and storing semen samples. There are limited options for fertility preservation for children and they currently involve ovarian tissue freezing, which is considered experimental. Nevertheless, there are options for adult female cancer patients to preserve their fertility.

Ovarian and Testicular Effects from Cancer Treatment

The ovary and testis are especially sensitive to chemotherapy. For women (and prepubertal girls), who have all been born with a finite number of oocytes (eggs), the reproductive impact from chemotherapy is contingent on the dose and type of therapy plus their age at treatment—younger patients are more likely to resist the damaging effects to the ovary. It is estimated that 40 percent of women younger than age 40 undergoing chemotherapy will experience ovarian failure following treatment. Certain chemotherapy drugs are more damaging to eggs than others (see table Chemotherapy Drugs Effect on Women on page 172); in the category of alkylating agents, the combination of oral CMF (cyclophosphamide, methotrexate, and fluorouracil), has the highest risk of ovarian failure following treatment. Posttherapy resumption of menses can occur in six months, but you may need to wait up to two years.

Radiation treatment for cancer can also impair fertility: Radiotherapy to the brain can disrupt signals to the ovary, disrupting ovulation and, if directed to the ovaries, creating the potential risk of inducing ovarian failure. Ovarian follicles are remarkably sensitive to DNA damage from radiation. A dose of above 300 cGy is the threshold for permanent ovarian failure. Most pelvic malignancies and Hodgkin lymphoma require radiation doses over 1,000 cGy and are associated with the highest risk for permanent loss of ovarian function.

It is important to note the return of menses does not mean a return to pretreatment biologic ovarian age. Cancer therapy results in the death of primordial (very early and immature) ovarian follicles and interrupts follicle maturation, resulting in decreasing ovarian reserve (number of eggs).

In men (and prepubertal boys), the testes are also susceptible to chemotherapy damage because this type of medication attacks rapidly dividing cells, such as sperm cells. Different from women, men begin making mature sperm following puberty. However, prepubertal sperm cells are at risk from chemotherapy damage as well.

As with females, radiotherapy can also have negative effects on reproduction: Radiotherapy to the brain can also disrupt vital signals to the testes for sperm and testosterone production; and directly to the testis can result in testicular failure depending on the dose of radiation.

Your reproductive potential following chemotherapy and radiation can still be impaired despite the return of menstrual cycles or the ability to ejaculate. Women, postchemotherapy, have a higher rate of infertility and lower ovarian reserve. Furthermore, even prior to therapy and for unexplained reasons, female cancer patients who pursue egg freezing for fertility preservation appear to have a reduced number of eggs retrieved compared with healthy controls of the same age.

CHEMOTHERAPY DRUGS EFFECT ON WOMEN	
HIGH RISK FOR EGG DAMAGE	LOW RISK FOR EGG DAMAGE
Busulfan	5-fluorouracil (5-FU)
Carboplatin	Bleomycin Sulfate
Carmustine (BCNU)	Cytarabine
Chlorambucil	Dactinomycin
Cisplatin	Daunorubicin Hydrochloride
Cyclophosphamide (Cytoxan)	Fludarabine Phosphate
Dacarbazine	Gemcitabine Hydrochloride
Doxorubicin (Adriamycin)	darubicin Hydrochloride
Ifosfamide	Methotrexate
Lomustine (CCNU)	Vinblastine Sulfate
Mechlorethamine Hydrochloride	Vincristine Sulfate

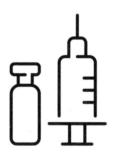

CHEMOTHERAPY DRUGS EFFECT ON MEN	
HIGH RISK FOR SPERM DAMAGE	LOW RISK FOR SPERM DAMAGE
Busulfan	5-fluorouracil (5-FU)
Carboplatin	6-Mercaptopurine (6-MP)
Carmustine	Bleomycin Sulfate
Chlorambucil	Cytarabine (Cytosar)
Cisplatin	Dacarbazine
Cyclophosphamide (Cytoxan®)	Daunorubicin Hydrochloride (Daunomycin)
Cytarabine	Doxorubicin Hydrochloride (Adriamycin)
Dactinomycin	Epirubicin Hydrochloride
Ifosfamide	Etoposide (VP-16)
Lomustine	Fludarabine Phosphate
Melphalan	Methotrexate
Mechlorethamine Hydrochloride	Mitoxantrone Hydrochloride

If you have lost your fertility potential because of chemotherapy and/or radiation, you can consider donor eggs, donor sperm, or adoption as options to achieve parenthood.

Ways to Preserve Your Fertility Prior to Cancer Treatment

The pendulum has swung to and fro regarding the effectiveness of a monthly GnRH agonist injection to preserve ovarian function. Remember in chapter 12: Endometriosis: Pain or Infertility? we talked about GnRH agonist. GnRH is produced in a top hormone stimulating center of the brain called the hypothalamus. GrRH agonist acts like GnRH to induce a "medical menopause," that is, the ovaries shut down since signals from the brain's pituitary are shut down. How does GnRH agonist protect your ovaries from chemotherapy? Well, we're not sure, but it does increase a protein called sphingosine-1-PO4 that protects immature eggs.

Bottom Line: There is no consensus among medical articles demonstrating any definitive benefit of using GnRH agonist for fertility preservation. Clinicians should still discuss the option with patients.

IVF with Embryo/Egg Freezing and Sperm Freezing

As a field, we have come far in broadening the indications of IVF. Now, we can provide a newly diagnosed cancer patient an "emergency" IVF for embryo or egg freezing. Because of an ovulation inhibitor called GnRH antagonist, we can begin stimulating a woman any day in her cycle and can usually complete the process within two weeks. This major advance make IVF easier in fertility preservation and reduces scheduling challenges for patients by using a random cycle day stimulation start rather than starting while on her menses. The antagonist can be initiated during injectable ovarian stimulation with immediate blockage from an ovulation risk as opposed to the two weeks needed for the same effect using the prior method, namely, GnRH agonist.

The technique for egg or embryo freezing has advanced over the last 10 years and uses a process called vitrification. This method has replaced the prior and cumbersome slow-freeze method. Most importantly, the more rapid freezing method of vitrification avoids the damaging ice crystal formation that can occur from slow freezing a woman's egg due to its high-water content. Consequently, pregnancy success rates with a vitrification–frozen embryo transfer or frozen egg cycle have significantly improved.

You can be encouraged that pregnancy outcomes of egg freezing are improving and nearing similar results as using fresh eggs. A report on the safety of egg freezing shows no increase in birth defects in 900 babies born from thawed eggs when compared to naturally conceived infants. Because the American Society for Reproductive Medicine, in 2012, lifted the experimental label on egg freezing, you can obtain this fertility preservation option at many IVF centers around the world.

Sperm freezing has existed for decades, long before egg freezing. Like eggs, sperm can be frozen for an indefinite time and thawing has not impaired pregnancy success.

Ovarian and Testicular Tissue Freezing (Experimental)

Ovarian tissue freezing by vitrification involves the surgical removal (via laparoscopy) of a portion of your ovary followed by freezing the tissue for later potential reimplantation into you in hope of restoring ovarian hormonal and ovulation function. This surgery is a low-risk outpatient procedure and requires minimal or no postponement of cancer treatment. Reimplantation of thawed ovarian tissue has led to the resumption of reproductive function and live births in cancer patients over the past decade. If this wasn't exciting enough, live births have occurred following a new combined approach of maturing the immature eggs from the surgically removed ovarian tissue. So stay tuned!

Testicular sperm freezing has been applied in a similar manner to ovarian tissue freezing and is very early in its application to help cancer patients prior to treatment.

Radiation Shielding and Ovarian or Testicular Protection

Pelvic radiation is commonly used in patients with cervical, vaginal, colorectal, and Hodgkin disease. To reduce radiation exposure to reproductive organs, lead shielding has traditionally been placed over the pelvis for a woman's ovaries and the genitals for a man's testes. When shielding is not possible, transposition (surgically moving) of ovaries away from the focus of the radiation field is used. There is variable success of ovarian function returning after surgical transposition (16 percent to 90 percent) due to either radiation effects, movement of the ovaries back to their original position, and damage to the ovarian blood supply. Several natural live births have occurred but most patients with transposed ovaries will require IVF to conceive. Because the ovaries have been moved out of the radiation focus of the pelvis, we perform egg retrieval placing a needle through your abdomen, rather than the vagina, with ultrasound guidance.

Following transposition, IVF live birth rates mainly depend on your age and the receptivity of your uterus (how likely an embryo will implant). Radiation to the uterus results in decreased implantation and increased rates of miscarriage. If you have had significant radiation damage to your uterus or if you have had a hysterectomy for definitive cancer therapy, you will require an IVF gestational carrier for your embryo transfer. Most recently, for women who have no uterus from either birth or hysterectomy, uterine transplantation is being offered. This is clearly considered experimental given only a few centers in the world are helping patients in this manner. Once another woman donates her uterus (donor), a surgery is necessary to implant the donor uterus into the recipient who experiences a prolonged hospitalization while being placed on immunosuppressant drugs to prevent rejection of the uterus. After one year on the immunosuppressant medications, the recipient will undergo IVF for conception—she cannot conceive naturally because the transplant does not include the fallopian tubes. She has the option of one or two pregnancies that must be delivered by cesarean section surgery for delivery of the baby. Once childbearing is complete, she will then undergo a subsequent hysterectomy to discontinue immunosuppressant drugs. Uterine transplantation is clearly in its infancy as an option for woman without a uterus to carry a pregnancy.

Testicular transposition can also be performed, like ovarian, to avoid the radiation focus but is not commonly used.

FERTILITY-SPARING OPTIONS FOR WOMEN	
STANDARD OF CARE	EXPERIMENTAL
Egg or embryo freezing	GnRH agonist
Conservative surgery	Ovarian tissue freezing
Moving the ovaries (Transposition)	Reimplant ovary (Orthotopic transplant)

FERTILITY-SPARING OPTIONS FOR MEN	
STANDARD OF CARE	EXPERIMENTAL
Sperm freezing	Testicular tissue freezing
Shielding the testes	Moving the testes (Transposition)

In Conclusion

Following treatment of your cancer, the optimal timing of a subsequent pregnancy will depend on your prognosis, your age, and your personal plans. All women who experience the devastation of a cancer diagnosis must be given fertility preservation options and be proactive in optimizing their subsequent ability to have a family.

CHAPTER 22
LGBTQ Fertility Options

Jeremy and Claus are a middle-aged gay male couple living in France and desiring a baby. In their country, sperm and egg donation are permitted but only with fully anonymous, altruistic donors; surrogacy is illegal. So they called our office to arrange a video consultation. Their request was IVF surrogacy using frozen eggs inseminated and fertilized so they both have the potential to be a biologic father. In other words, if they purchase 8 mature frozen eggs, then they would like 4 inseminated by each of their sperm samples. They had one more request—a double embryo transfer, which means two embryos, one fertilized by each of them.

Especially since we are using an egg donor, we recommend the number of embryos to transfer be consistent with ASRM guidelines. There are clearly two sides to this couple's request. One is the medical concern that a twin pregnancy is high risk but the other is the financial concern that two single pregnancy gestational carrier cycles costs in the tens of thousands of dollars. I believe my obligation is to educate and provide the best medical evidence-based care so patients can make an informed decision. After considering all risks, patients have the right to informed refusal, meaning they understand the risks and would like to proceed against medical recommendations.

In 1996, while nearing the completion of my fellowship in reproductive endocrinology, I began applying for positions where I would practice my specialty. During one of my interviews, the senior physician of the practice asked how I felt about single women. I lightheartedly reminded him I was married, even though I knew the real reason for his question—would I treat single women or lesbian couples with donor sperm to conceive.

Trying to be diplomatic in a conservative hospital, I respectfully—but clearly—expressed my passion for treating all those who are having difficulty conceiving a baby, whether they are a heterosexual married or unmarried couple, single woman, or lesbian/gay couple. His argument on why I should reconsider my position was not only futile but insulting when he asked, "Would you want a woman marching in a gay pride parade wearing a T-shirt with the statement, 'Dr. Trolice helped me have my baby?'" Without any hesitation, I shot back, "Yes. Would you rather have her T-shirt say, 'Dr. Trolice refused to help me have a baby?'" He was unable to respond—I made my point.

More than twenty years after that uncomfortable yet liberating exchange, LGBTQ patients continue to face unnecessary social obstacles along their road to parenthood—all due to prejudice. I think you'd all agree that prejudice in any form has caused indelible consequences in our world and cripples our progress as a civilized society. Yet it continues to pervade and infect all aspects of our lives. Unfortunately, medicine is not immune to discrimination, such as the way some patients are treated who are morbidly obese, indigent, LGBTQ, and still due to their race and religion. This chapter will focus on LGBTQ patients to empower that community with fertility options as well as educate all readers.

Reproductive Options for Lesbian Couples or Single Women

As lesbians and single women, you all have the option to conceive with the use of donor sperm either through vaginal, otherwise called intracervical insemination (ICI), or IUI with donor sperm. ICI involves depositing the sperm at the opening of the cervix as opposed to entering the uterine cavity as with IUI.

Attempting to conceive with donor sperm, you have two options: using sperm either from an anonymous or from a known donor. Either option should employ FDA guidelines requiring STI testing and a frozen quarantine of sperm from a nonintimate partner: seven days of freezing for a known sperm donor; and six months of freezing for an anonymous donor. Fortunately, with the use of frozen-thawed sperm, there has not been a reported case of an STI. To locate a sperm bank in the United States, you can visit SpermBankDirectory.com for a directory. To locate a sperm bank from practically anywhere in the world, visit the Global IVF website at globalivf.com/directory/services/sperm-banks.

Prior to treatment, we will evaluate your medical and reproductive history, perform a physical exam, test you for ovulation function, and obtain blood work for a pre-pregnancy health screen. Additionally, we can determine if there are any abnormalities that may interfere with conception by offering a pelvic ultrasound and an HSG to determine tubal patency (whether there are any blockages or adhesions involving your fallopian tubes). The ASRM strongly recommends you undergo a psychological counseling session if you are planning to use a sperm, egg, or embryo donor. The session is meant as a comprehensive education and consent process for you to address the unique form of reproduction.

Once the evaluation is complete, you can simply use a home OPK that detects your pituitary LH surge in the urine that triggers ovulation. Once the OPK turns positive, a single IUI procedure can be performed the same or next day, as opposed to two days in a row (one IUI procedure per ovulation has the same pregnancy rate as two).

The cumulative pregnancy rate observed in up to 12 insemination cycles was 74 percent if you are younger than 31 years, decreases to 62 percent if you are aged 31 to 35 years, and to 54 percent if you are older than 35 years.

Following at least six unsuccessful cycles, if you are older than 35 years, we can discuss hormonal treatments as part of your insemination cycle to increase the number of eggs (oocytes) released per ovulation to potentially improve the pregnancy rate. Fertility medication will also increase the risk of a multiple pregnancy (as reviewed in chapter 21: Early Pregnancy Complications), so caution not to greatly exceed risk is key.

The method of insemination does appear to influence the outcome. In single women undergoing donor sperm insemination, placing the sperm intrauterine results in a higher live birth rate rather than depositing the sperm inside the cervix. The monthly fertility rate for IUI is approximately 15 percent, as compared with 9 percent for ICI in single women without known fertility problems. There appear to be no clinical studies comparing IUI with depositing the sperm inside the entrance of the vagina using a syringe.

Ultimately, if IUI is not successful, IVF may be necessary for you to conceive. In lesbian couples, egg sharing is a unique option and depends on the partner's egg quality and quantity. One partner may choose to share her eggs with the other partner so she can carry the pregnancy. Through the advanced reproductive technology of IVF, the partner providing the eggs would be stimulated with hormones and have her eggs harvested. Her eggs would then be fertilized with donor sperm, followed by embryo transfer into her partner's uterine cavity that had been prepared by hormones to optimize implantation.

Gay Male Couples or Single Men

The converse to single women and lesbian couples, men desiring children not only lack an egg source but also a uterus to carry the pregnancy. The number of gay male couples desiring biological parenthood by requiring an egg donor and a gestational carrier continues to grow globally.

Through the services of egg donation, either fresh or frozen eggs, and GCs, you can now utilize IVF to achieve a successful pregnancy.

Single men and gay male couples desiring a biologically related child require the services of an egg donor who provides the eggs as well as a GC. This process may occur through traditional surrogacy or an IVF GC. Traditional surrogacy is when the woman who will carry the pregnancy also is the source of the egg. She usually will ovulate naturally and undergo IUI. Very few, if any, infertility clinics offer traditional surrogacy as states vary in their laws overseeing this arrangement, so it is imperative that, in advance of your treatment cycle, you consult with an attorney who is well versed in this area.

IVF GC is the process of using an egg donor and a separate carrier.

Following hormonal stimulation of the egg donor and egg retrieval, the eggs are fertilized with the sperm of one or both partners in a reproductive laboratory through IVF. Your embryo is then transferred into the GC's uterus, previously prepared hormonally to synchronize optimal receptivity. The resulting baby is genetically unrelated to the carrier.

Transgender Men

In 2017 a transgender man named Patrick (not his real name) and his girlfriend came into to my office wanting to have a baby. Being genetically female with ovaries, the man wanted me to harvest his eggs, inseminate them with donor sperm, and transfer an embryo into his wife.

While the reproductive biology was simple, the psychosocial reality was profound—for all of us.

During our first consultation, Patrick was very anxious but determined. While I tried to place him and his girlfriend at ease by demonstrating our commitment to all fertility patients, Patrick became preoccupied and was not forthcoming with his concern. As we completed the conversation, I recommended an examination and pelvic ultrasound to assess Patrick's ovarian age as an indicator for the number of eggs we would expect to harvest. After the physical exam, I asked Patrick to place his legs in the stirrups, so I could insert the vaginal probe ultrasound—he looked devastated. It was then I learned his preoccupation.

For years, Patrick assumed the life of a man. He had undergone bilateral mastectomy and hormonal therapy using testosterone to appear masculine—which he did. Standing in front of him, I finally realized the reason for his anguish. By performing a pelvic ultrasound, I would be reminding Patrick of his internal female anatomy. And what was worse, he would be showing his ovaries to his girlfriend.

My sensitivity and compassion for this wonderful couple accelerated to the highest level. Patrick loved his girlfriend more than his embarrassment of revealing his ovaries. His girlfriend loved him more than his genetics. Together they would be my first transgender male and female couple. I was honored to assist them and overjoyed when they had their baby.

Transgender Patients

A transgender female is born genetically male, so provided her external genitalia are not surgically altered and her hormone therapy has not impaired sperm production, she can impregnate her female partner through sexual intercourse. Other options include preparation of sperm for IUI into their designated female partner, if applicable, or a GC.

Of importance, fertility preservation is a valuable option for transgender patients to provide their eggs and sperm prior to hormonal or surgical transition. Eggs can be harvested and frozen while sperm can be obtained through ejaculation for freezing. Fortunately frozen eggs and sperm have no current biologic time limit. Following fertility preservation, patients can proceed with the transgender transition.

Adoption

In 2013, same-sex parents in the United States were four times more likely than different-sex parents to be raising an adopted child. (The Williams Institute UCLA School of Law reports that among couples with children under the age of 18 in the home, 13 percent of same-sex parents have an adopted child, compared to just 3 percent of different-sex parents.)

As the number of same-sex parents continued to rise and more states made same-sex parental adoption legal, a federal judge ruled in 2016 that Mississippi's ban on same-sex couples who desire to adopt children was unconstitutional, thereby making gay adoption legal in all 50 states.

Then, in 2017, the United States heralded another breakthrough when the Supreme Court reversed an Arkansas Supreme Court ruling and ordered all 50 states to treat same-sex couples equally to opposite-sex couples in the issuance of birth certificates.

Around the world, many other countries do allow adoption by same-sex couples; however, some countries do require the couples to be married prior to adoption.

Equality?

Upon recognizing that its nondiscrimination state laws were being violated by restricting fertility coverage solely to heterosexual married couples, California became the first state to enact a law that ensures unmarried and gay couples have the same access to insurance coverage for fertility treatments as heterosexual married couples. That was in 2013.

Since then, no other state has yet to repeat what California accomplished. True, seven other states have since taken action to expand infertility treatments beyond heterosexual married couples, their successes have been limited.

However, all this occurred before the WHO decided to consider revising its definition of infertility. Under the proposed revision, which went out to national health ministers in 2017, a person who wants to become a parent doesn't have to be in a sexual relationship—or one that could lead to a pregnancy—to qualify as "infertile."

Such a decision would be significant in that it would lead to policy changes worldwide.

With their new definition, the WHO could finally open the door for increasing equality with respect to infertility treatment and insurance coverage on a global scale.

While we have yet to see what the WHO will decide, 2017 was proven to be an uptick in United States legislative activity on the subject. For example, as I write this chapter, a group of LGBTQ activists in Hawaii is pushing for legislation that would require insurance companies to cover IVF for more couples, including making Hawaii the first state to require such coverage for gestational carriers, which would help male same-sex couples who must use a GC. (While laws vary among states, all patients pursuing third-party reproduction should engage a reproductive health attorney in order to protect all those involved.)

In Conclusion

Gradually, the United States and the rest of the world are changing their laws to allow more reproductive rights for nonheterosexual patients. However, there is still much work to be accomplished.

Reproductive technology now allows more family building options for the LGBTQ community than ever before. Whether by IUI, IVF, gestational carrier, donor egg, or donor sperm, as long as there is no medical contraindication, legal, or ethical restriction to provide treatment, it all comes down to the core belief that every person and couple deserve fertility care. Thankfully this belief is being embraced, albeit slowly, in the United States and around the world.

CHAPTER 23

Three Case Histories on Donation and Adoption

We are defined by the choices we make and our outlook on life. All of us begin with dreams of our ideal existence though, invariably, adjustments are a necessity. Whether we support a fatalist philosophy or believe in God's plan, one thing is certain—no one's life matches our original design.

As a fertility patient, ironically, your most significant challenge to overcome is not the decision of which treatment option to pursue, or even the mounting expense of tests and therapy. For many, your obstacle is both simple and complicated: shame. Of all the medical diseases with their associated treatment, infertility patients' responses to their diagnosis contradict all other medical approaches to resolution. Consider a newly diagnosed cancer patient internally bargaining to avoid surgery, chemotherapy, and/or radiation and determined to heal naturally. Yet many infertility patients reject or delay medical assistance for that exact reason.

The ability to conceive, for centuries, has represented the ultimate accomplishment of our species in the strictest evolutionary terms. Women often express their procreative prowess with pride and define the duration of time to conceive as the benchmark of their femininity. Many men define their fertility as the extreme representation of their virility. These interpretations are clearly unjustified but perpetuate the stigma of infertility and explain a patient's guilt, isolation, and embarrassment.

Why would the initiation of infertility treatment denote failure in the minds of some of you? Certainly this reaction is inappropriate, but it is also unfair to you while enduring the emotional devastation of infertility and fearing a life of being childless. The feeling of shame can paralyze you and sabotage the path toward building a family. It is also responsible for secretive visits to the infertility specialist to withhold the struggle from even the closest family and friends.

For as difficult as infertility treatments may be, alternative options such as egg donation, sperm donation, embryo donation, and adoption can be the psychological apocalypse.

Here are some stories of real patients.

Case History 1: "I don't want anyone to know it's not a part of me."

Recently a delightful couple for whom I have been privileged to care, requested I withhold information about their use of egg donation from their obstetrician. My reply was reassuring: I would never reveal their treatment option without their approval. However, there was one problem—her advanced reproductive age would compel her physician to strongly recommend testing for chromosomal abnormalities, such as Down syndrome. Of course, the patient could refuse testing, but there was a more significant reason she offered for her request: "I don't want anyone to know it's not a part of me."

We had just completed her embryo transfer and the words resonated throughout the procedure room, transforming the silence to a distracting noise. Momentarily at a loss, I asked if I could share my thoughts. The room was quiet except for our ubiquitous Enya music in the background. As I struggled to find a sensitive approach employing science and psychology, while realizing her right to withhold the information, I was quickly and thankfully reminded that her story was my story, too.

Being raised in a northern New Jersey close-knit Italian circle, I learned and appreciated the importance of family. When infertility struck me, I experienced a myriad of confusing and overwhelming emotions. Following a decade of testing, treatment, and complications, we resolved our infertility through the blessing of adoption. Why ten years? Because our natural desire was not being realized and we stubbornly endured years of struggle simply for biology.

During that time, my wife and I endured every test, surgery, treatment cycle, and complication the disease can offer. Yet we were unable to build our family in the manner we planned.

The idea of adoption occurred to us intermittently but never prevailed until we moved to Florida. After my wife's last surgery, we jointly decided to end our infertility and proactively select an alternative path.

Five children later, my only regret is not having adopted in an earlier stage of our infertility to avoid the heartache—both financial and physical.

Nevertheless, any earlier adoption would have prevented us from knowing and being blessed with the angels we adore.

However, it comes as no astonishment that parents usually will effortlessly love their biologically related children. After all, how challenging is loving a true part of you? Not because biological parents are narcissists but take enormous pleasure in the accomplishment of creating life through the union with their partner. Hence the hurdle of accepting an alternative path to this original plan.

Yet what is biology? We accept the physical similarities biological children have with their parents as ingratiating. All children also inherit genetic risks of disease, for example, cancer, diabetes, and cardiovascular problems. Of importance, there is no definitive certainty children will be endowed with the special talents and traits of their biological parents. After all, do any of us recall Einstein's, Pasteur's, or Mozart's offspring following in the footsteps of their eternally renowned parents?

Remarkably, our emerging understanding of epigenetics allows a biologic phenomenon—namely, environmental factors that turn certain genes on or off. Consequently, nurture meets nature in facilitating the potential genetic influence by adoptive parents to allow their nonbiologically related children the potential to inherit certain familial traits.

The gift of life presents in many forms. When an infertility patient turns to nonbiologic options of family building, they dedicate themselves to the purest form of our existence, which is loving for the sake of love, without genetic strings.

Neither shame nor clandestine behavior ever should emerge from this magnanimous and beneficent act. Rather, the new parent can confidently relish in the adjustment of their plan and enjoy all the joy, fulfillment, and love that parenting offers.

I was not informed whether she shared use of an egg donor with her OB/GYN, but her words will always remain with me: "It's not a part of me." Quite the contrary. This gift of life has been deliberately chosen and defines the very nature of our being.

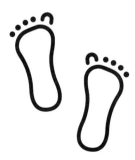

Case History 2: "My ankles have always been swollen."

Rarely in a lifetime, let alone a medical career, can one person truly affect another person in a profound way. Even more unique is when two people share in the joy of enlightenment.

Fortunately, two such memorable events happened with me.

Having a typical day in the office, I was called by my receptionist and asked if I would be able to see an unscheduled patient who was not infertile or interested in having children until next year but had been told she had PCOS. Since I was available and thought this would be a simple consultation, I agreed to see her.

We began by discussing Marie's frustration over her symptoms: a long history of irregular menses, pelvic discomfort, and acne. Feeling experienced in PCOS, I provided Marie the explanation of why PCOS caused her problems and how we could help alleviate them. Marie complained, "All doctors just tell me to take the birth control pill, but it's not helping any longer." After 20 minutes, Marie shared her burden of significant stress over turning 30 years of age, starting her own business, and planning to be married . . . all within a year! Not surprisingly, her symptoms had all been worsening. When I raised this coincidence to Marie, she was relieved to realize stress may be the culprit in causing all her troubling symptoms that were previously being managed by the BCP. I then offered to examine Marie to confirm my diagnosis but was quite proud of myself for making this connection for her. However, my hubris proved to be faulty.

The exam was entirely normal and, unexpectedly, she had no evidence of dark hair growth in the usual areas of PCOS women. Toward the end of the physical and because she was on BCPs, I examined and asked about her legs to ensure there was no evidence of a rare blood clot. This is when Marie casually conveyed, "My ankles have always been swollen." When I asked her to elaborate, she explained her swelling has been present ever since she was a dancer.

It is not an exaggeration when I describe my feeling as a paralysis. Had I not examined her legs and she not offered the history of swollen ankles, I would not have learned she suffered from the Female Athlete Triad. She further added that, as a competitive dancer, she developed bulimia (a condition where a person self-induces vomiting following meals).

The Female Athlete Triad consists of amenorrhea (lack of menstruation), energy deficit (from inadequate caloric intake as can occur with an eating disorder), and bone loss (from the ovaries not producing estrogen due to a disruption of brain signals).

Anorexia/bulimia has a 5 to 15 percent mortality rate, and up to 30 percent of women remain with ovulation dysfunction despite recovery.

As a physician, I had been taught that if you give the patient enough time, she will tell you the cause of her problem. Knowing the true origin of her symptoms and her new diagnosis, Marie was overwhelmed and relieved. She never shared this history with any prior physician and my revelation was clearly serendipitous.

After I educated her on her diagnosis, she appeared determined to correct her calorie deficit. We scheduled her to see a nutritionist and she agreed to reduce her exercise to no more than a moderate level of exertion.

As she left the office with more hope than when she arrived, she thanked me for helping her, but I expressed my gratitude to her for reminding me why I embrace the art of medicine and how privileged I am to care for patients.

Case History 3: "The risk you do not pursue."

Before telling you about one more of my most memorable moments with a patient, let me preface the story by saying that we all need to be intermittently reminded of our purpose throughout our lives.

Working in IVF, I share in some of the happiest and some of the saddest moments in a patient's life. While trying to help create a life, I am continually reminded that success is not a guarantee. My goal has always been to provide my maximum medical effort for every woman/man/couple with whom I have the privilege to work. This next experience taught me to persevere, even when medicine fails.

While sitting in an ultrasound exam room filled with hope for signs of a new life, Rachel and Adriel awaited the outcome from years of infertility and treatments.

Following a brief sharing of her symptoms, an uncomfortable silence enveloped the room as Rachel prepared for a vaginal ultrasound to determine if her pregnancy was viable.

Rachel's and Adriel's eyes were fixed on the ultrasound monitor. They had been down this road before. Infertility had consumed their marriage, and they had just completed their final IVF attempt. Five weeks earlier, we thawed and transferred their last remaining embryo. Now years of struggle became defined by one moment in time.

Many patients have passed through my office. Each with a unique story, but all with the same purpose—a healthy baby. As a physician, I've lived their stories for over 20 years, including my own prolonged, arduous road as an infertility patient. My privilege and honor are being part of another's profound life-altering journey.

As they held their breaths, Rachel and Adriel braced for my diagnosis. The ultrasound was obvious, and I softly conveyed to them, "I'm sorry but you've lost another baby." Their world began to crumble in front of me. They were totally silent with despair. No tears. Only their stoic, expressionless acceptance. As they left my office, I felt their pain and a personal sense of failure.

All at once, given their ages and journey, I was reminded of how my wife and I endured years of unsuccessful fertility treatment. Because of our blessings with adoption, we established and ran our own adoption agency for several years. Subsequent to closing the agency, my wife continued to receive notices of babies available for placement, which we had routinely referred to friends, acquaintances, and patients interested in expanding their families.

With destiny in the air, another adoption notice arrived for my wife on the very evening of Rachel's and Adriel's loss. Following the tragedy of a miscarriage, it's important for couples to grieve to resolve their loss. Having known Rachel and Adriel for some time, I considered gently sharing with them the news of a potential baby for adoption. Later that same evening, upon hearing the news, Rachel's tears turned to laughter. I provided the necessary contact information and I prayed for them to be selected by the birth giver.

Over the next three months, my wife guided Rachel and Adriel through the necessary steps toward adoption. We received welcome updates regularly and were overjoyed when we learned they were accepted to be the adopting parents.

The day they brought their daughter home was three months to the day after their last pregnancy loss.

No one's life proceeds according to plan—one door closes, another opens. Rachel and Adriel chose to walk through the newly opened door because they realized the only regret in life is, the risk you do not pursue.

In Conclusion

The best definition of stress I have heard is "trying to control something you cannot." Infertility is not something you can control. Acceptance is a huge part of the infertility journey—not to resign from having children, but to be open to advanced reproductive treatment and alternative methods that may hopefully fill your home with the joy you have been anticipating.

CHAPTER 24

The Top Ten Questions and the Hard Facts about Each

1. What is the definition of infertility?

The World Health Organization (WHO) defines infertility as "a disease of the reproductive system defined by the failure to achieve a clinical pregnancy after 12 months or more of regular unprotected sexual intercourse." In the United States, the accepted definition includes "without predisposing risk factors" such as age, medical, sexual and reproductive history, physical findings, and diagnostic testing. As a global health issue, infertility affects 10 percent of women worldwide.

The monthly rate of natural conception for women less than age 30 without fertility problems is only 20 percent, but after one year, approximately 85 percent of these couples will have conceived. Compare this to age 40 where the monthly natural pregnancy rate is only 5 percent.

2. What are the most common reasons for infertility in heterosexual couples?

At your first visit with me, I share with you that the purpose of an infertility evaluation is to hopefully find an area to correct and never to find a reason to blame. If a couple love each other enough to bring a life into this world and their home, then they are strong enough to approach any cause of their problem as one step closer to hopefully having a baby together.

An infertility evaluation should be efficient and thorough to expedite your time to treatment. Your physician should validate your concerns and provide evidence-based, researched options toward your goal.

During testing, factors can be identified as potentially contributing to the cause of your infertility. The approximate breakdown is as follows:

- Female factors—40 percent (further divided by ovulation disorders in 40 percent and tubal disease in 40 percent)
- Male factors—40 percent
- Unexplained factors—20 percent.
- Combination of factors to be determined (30 percent)

3. What are fertility medications and how do they work?

Fertility medications are simply drugs that help you conceive. The most common fertility medications are classified as ovulation induction drugs and have been FDA approved for patients with ovulation disorders. When a woman has ovulation dysfunction, the goal of these medications is to allow the woman to produce one to two ovarian follicular cysts (follicles) to ovulate (release the egg[s]).

These medications can also be prescribed even if you ovulate in order to make you "super" ovulate, that is, release more than one egg from the ovary at the time of ovulation.

Bypassing the usual female hormonal pathways of the brain and ovary, these medications stimulate the ovary to produce more than the typical one follicle with an egg per month. When more eggs are produced, more are potentially exposed to sperm, thereby increasing the chance for pregnancy.

Oral fertility medications are clomiphene citrate (Clomid, Serophene) and letrozole (Femara), the use of which usually results in one or two follicles each cycle; they occasionally result in three or more follicles, thereby increasing the risk of multiples. Clomiphene citrate was first approved for medical use in 1967. Letrozole, though not approved for ovulation induction, has become the first-line medication for those of you with PCOS.

The other class of drugs are all called gonadotropins (Menopur, Follistim, Gonal-F) and are currently administered by injection. They mimic the normal brain signals to stimulate the ovary to produce many mature follicles each cycle. In ovulatory patients, these medications should be combined with IUI or can be used during IVF.

4. Why would I need a laparoscopy?

Your gynecologist will have you undergo testing to determine the possible cause of infertility. Unfortunately, 20 percent of couples experience unexplained infertility. Although unexplained infertility has traditionally only been diagnosed following a laparoscopic surgery, I do not recommend undergoing this procedure if your HSG and pelvic ultrasound are both normal and you have no concerning symptoms for endometriosis, namely, chronic severe painful periods (dysmenorrhea) and painful intercourse (dyspareunia).

Laparoscopy is an outpatient same-day operative procedure and involves insertion of a telescope through your belly button into your abdomen to view your internal pelvic reproductive organs, while you are under general anesthesia. This procedure will allow a definite diagnosis of pelvic adhesions, tubal scarring or blockage, endometriosis, or other abnormalities that may negatively impact your fertility.

In the infertility world, laparoscopy is limited to the evaluation and treatment of

- Hydrosalpinges (blocked and dilated ends of your fallopian tubes)
- Removal of a uterine cavity distorting fibroid (often using a robotic device)
- Suspected endometriosis based on severely painful periods, painful intercourse, and/or a probable endometrioma (ovarian "chocolate" cyst of endometriosis)
- Ovarian drilling to surgically induce ovulation in women with PCOS (See chapter 13: Polycystic Ovary Syndrome [PCOS].)
- Tubal reversal surgery to open fallopian tubes in women who have undergone a sterilization procedure called bilateral tubal ligation (tying off and blocking the tubes)

While laparoscopy used to be part of every fertility evaluation, medical evidence tells us there is limited to no value of this procedure to try and diagnose a cause of your infertility if you have a normal HSG and pelvic ultrasound. This surgery should not be offered as part of a routine evaluation of unexplained infertility when your HSG and pelvic ultrasound are both normal and you have no concerning symptoms for endometriosis, as described above and in chapter 12.

5. What is an HSG (hysterosalpingogram)?

During an evaluation for infertility, 40 percent of female factors are due to tubal blockage. First performed in the early 20th century to assess the fallopian tubes, an HSG is occurs in an office or hospital during which X-rays are taken while contrast dye is instilled through the cervix into the uterus and fallopian tubes. The procedure is usually brief and associated with mild to moderate uterine cramping depending on the experience of the physician and your anatomy. You are awake and can often watch the monitor with your physician to see the results of the study.

6. What is intrauterine insemination (IUI)?

IUI is the use of partner or donor sperm for insemination. It can be performed during a nonmedicated cycle (natural cycle) or a cycle stimulated by fertility medications. There are only a few indications for natural cycle IUI:

- The couple are unable to have or complete intercourse.
- The man has retrograde ejaculation, where sperm enters the bladder at the time of ejaculation. The treatment is to recover sperm by urination following orgasm and ejaculation, process the sperm in the lab, then proceed with IUI.
- The woman is using donor sperm.

Live birth rates from IUI treatment cycles vary, but studies have demonstrated a rate of approximately 10% per month.

My patients often worry that IUI increases the risk for a multiple pregnancy, but only fertility medications increase the number of eggs that ovulate with the resulting higher chance for twins (< 5 percent for oral meds and < 20 percent for gonadotropins) and, rarely, triplets or higher (< 1 percent for oral meds and < 5 percent for gonadotropins).

IUI involves washing the semen sample remove chemicals from the semen and separate the sperm from the semen. The actual preparation of the sperm sample enhances its fertilization potential. The sample of sperm is concentrated to a small volume that contains the highest number of moving sperm and then placed into your uterus by passing a small plastic catheter through the cervix. This is a brief and minor office procedure that is usually associated with minimal to no discomfort. The processing of the sperm stimulates fertilization potential and the procedure places a large concentration of moving sperm into the upper uterus, thereby decreasing the distance to the fallopian tubes where they travel to fertilize an egg.

Of note, ejaculated sperm *must* be processed in the manner described above prior to IUI; otherwise, you will experience a severe reaction of uterine contractions because seminal fluid have chemicals caused prostaglandins.

7. What is the relationship between fertility and age?

This is *the* question to consider when TTC. No matter what an ovarian test results show, your birthday is the best predictor of success. Why? Because you are born with all the eggs you will ovulate in your lifetime. Until puberty, all your eggs are resting at a certain stage of development. Beginning with your first period (menarche), hundreds of eggs are stimulated each month, but only one egg will typically complete development and ovulate, the rest will regress. If you are 25 years old, then you have 25-year-old eggs; at 35 years of age, your eggs are also 35.

As you age, the number and quality of your eggs diminishes. This explains the studies of women demonstrating a consistent decline in fertility beginning around age 30. Accordingly, your monthly pregnancy rates based on age are as follows on the next page.

YOUR AGE	MONTHLY NATURAL PREGNANCY RATE
30	20%
35	10%
40	5%

There is a more marked decline in fertility after age 40 due to older eggs that are less responsive eggs to your brain's and medication stimulation. If this isn't bad enough, as you get older, there is an increase in miscarriage—from 10 percent at age under 30 to 33 percent at age 40—usually caused by genetic abnormalities of the embryo.

Age can also affect men in terms of sexual function, frequency of sexual relations and sperm production. For men over age 40, recent evidence supports an increase in infertility, miscarriage, preterm birth, and the child's risk for autism, schizophrenia, chromosomal abnormalities, and birth defects.

8. What is the workup for the male?

Since 40 percent of infertile heterosexual couples will have a male factor, it is imperative for us to evaluate the male. The initial workup will include obtaining your medical history to investigate any potential areas that could be contributing to infertility. While there is no definitive fertility test (outside of pregnancy) to demonstrate the ability of your sperm to fertilize an egg, the best screen is the comprehensive SA.

The SA examines collected sperm and reports on a number of parameters, most importantly count (density), percent moving (motility), and percent with normal shapes (morphology). Based on these results, we make a recommendation to proceed with further testing by a urologist, preferably one who specializes in male infertility.

9. What is in vitro fertilization (IVF)?

IVF is an ART procedure whereby fertilization of the eggs and sperm occur in the laboratory. The cycle usually begins with an ultrasound and hormonal testing while you are on your period. Next you begin to self-administer daily injectable fertility medications (gonadotropins, discussed previously) to stimulate multiple follicle cyst toward producing multiple mature eggs. Over the course of 10 days, on average, you will visit your fertility clinic every 2 to 4 days for ultrasound measurements of your follicles and hormonal blood testing, so your physician can adjust your medication accordingly based on your response. When the ovarian follicles measure the appropriate size, you will receive instructions for a trigger injection, so the eggs can mature inside the follicles. Approximately 36 hours following the trigger, you will be scheduled for your egg-retrieval procedure, which is under intravenous conscious sedation and usually in an office-based surgery center.

The egg-retrieval procedure involves placing a needle through the vagina into the ovary under ultrasound guidance for multiple follicle cyst aspiration. Timing is everything here! Once you receive the trigger injection, the clock starts. If you wait more than 38 to 40 hours from the trigger injection, the eggs may spontaneous release or ovulate resulting in a canceled cycle due to lost eggs.

During the retrieval, your eggs are identified by the embryologist in the lab.

Approximately four to six hours later, sperm are added for fertilization. The following day, we notify you how many embryos (fertilized eggs) developed.

Once embryos are formed, multiple options ensue, based on your individual situation:

- Freeze all embryos (unless this was an egg freezing cycle)
- Monitor growth for transfer on day three or five
- Biopsy the embryos on day five or six for PGT-A and/or PGT-M

Live births from IVF are typically based on the woman's age but can be influenced by day of embryo transfer and the use of fresh versus frozen embryos. Valuable sites for national and clinic specific outcomes are available at sart.org and cdc.gov/art. The key is to have your IVF cycle personalized to meet your specific reproductive problem and have your clinical/laboratory team ready, on a daily basis, to adjust the plan accordingly based on developments.

10. When should I be referred to a fertility specialist?

This is an excellent question and one that is very individualized depending, most importantly, on your diagnosis, female age, motivation level, and financial resources.

In general, after the gynecologist has performed an initial workup, the patient and the gynecologist should devise a plan and timeline after which referral should be recommended to a board-certified REI specialist. There is evidence that an earlier referral to a specialist shortens the time to pregnancy.

There are some situations where a patient should be referred immediately to a fertility specialist:

- Advanced reproductive age above 39
- Irregular or no periods
- Blocked fallopian tubes
- Severe Male Factor

Most importantly, your physician should refer you to a specialist based on *your* desire to accelerate the process to an advanced evaluation and more treatment options.

In Conclusion

These 10 topics essentially summarize my purpose of this book—to know how long you should allow natural attempts at conception; to know an evidence based infertility evaluation; to know appropriate treatment options and their realistic success rates; and to know you are in charge.

An REI specialist is, in my opinion, the best GPS you can have. Think of being in your car in need of directions. The GPS provides guidance, gives you options for faster routes, but you decide on the path.

My prayer for you all is this book has become your GPS to empower you along your journey. You are all my Fertility Warriors and have endured more heartache than your peers regarding reproduction, but you've gained valuable insight into your tenacity and courage.

May your arms and hearts be forever full of the love you seek today.

Definitions of Acronyms and Initialisms

ACRONYM/INITIALISM	FULL NAME
ABOG	American Board of Obstetrics and Gynecology
ACOG	American College of Obstetricians and Gynecologists
AFC	antral follicle count
AMA	advanced maternal age
AMH	Anti-Müllerian hormone
APA	antiphospholipid antibodies
APS	antiphospholipid syndrome
ARC	Advanced Reproductive Care, Inc
ART	assisted reproductive technology
ASRM	American Society for Reproductive Medicine
BBT	basal body temperature
BCP	birth control pill
BMI	body mass index
CBAVD	congenital bilateral absence of the vas deferens
CCCT	clomiphene citrate challenge test
CCS	comprehensive chromosome screening
CE	chronic endometritis
CRISPR	clustered regularly interspaced short palindromic repeats
CVS	chorionic villus sampling
DOR	diminished ovarian reserve

DS	Down syndrome
EFI	Endometriosis Fertility Index
EGA	estimated gestational age
ERA	endometrial receptivity assay
FET	frozen embryo transfer
FHR	fetal heart rate
FSH	follicle stimulating hormone
GC	gestational carrier
GnRH	gonadotropin-releasing hormone
GnRH agonist	gonadotropin-releasing hormone agonist
GnRH antagonist	gonadotropin-releasing hormone antagonist
hCG	human chorionic gonadotropin
HSG	hysterosalpingogram
ICI	intracervical insemination
ICSI	intracytoplasmic sperm injection
IP	intended parent
IUD	intrauterine device
IUI	intrauterine insemination
IUP	intrauterine pregnancy
IVF	in vitro fertilization
LH	luteinizing hormone
LOD	laparoscopic ovarian diathermy
MESA	microsurgical epididymal sperm aspiration
MIS	minimally invasive surgery
MRI	magnetic resonance imaging
NNT	number needed to treat

NOA	non-obstructive ozoospermia
OA	obstructive ozoospermia
OB/GYN	obstetrician/gynecologist or obstetrics/gynecology
OBD	oil-based dye
OHSS	ovarian hyperstimulation syndrome
OMD	Oriental Medicine Doctors
OPK	ovulation predictor kit
OSA	obstructive sleep apnea
PCOS	polycystic ovary syndrome
PGS	preimplantation genetic screening
PGT	preimplantation genetic testing
PGT-A	preimplantation genetic testing for aneuploidy
PGT-M	preimplantation genetic testing for monogenic disorders
PID	pelvic inflammatory disease
PNV	prenatal vitamin
POF	premature ovarian failure
PUL	pregnancy of unknown location
REI	reproduction endocrinology and infertility
RM	recurrent miscarriages
RPL	recurrent pregnancy loss
SA	semen analysis
SAA	salivary alpha-amylase
SART	Society for Assisted Reproductive Technology
SIS	saline infusion sonogram
SQ	subcutaneous
SREI	Society for Reproductive Endocrinology and Infertility

STI	sexually transmitted infection
TESA	testicular sperm aspiration
TFI	tubal factor infertility
TPO	thyroid peroxidase antibodies
TSH	thyroid-stimulating hormone
TTC	trying to conceive
TUVS	transvaginal ultrasound
TV	testicular volume
UPT	urine pregnancy test
WCD	water contrast dye
WHO	World Health Organization
YCMD	Y chromosome microdeletion

Resources

For additional information about fertility and infertility, visit the websites of the following organizations:

American Board of Obstetrics and Gynecology / abog.org

The American College of Obstetricians and Gynecologists / acog.org

American Society for Reproductive Medicine / asrm.org

ARC Fertility / arcfertility.com

European Society of Human Reproduction and Embryology / eshre.org

FertilityIQ / fertilityiq.com

The National Infertility Association / resolve.org

Path2Parenthood / path2parenthood.org

Reproductive Facts / reproductivefacts.org

Society for Assisted Reproductive Technology / sart.org

Society for Reproductive Endocrinology and Fertility / socrei.org

The Society of Reproductive Surgeons / reprodsurgery.org

About the Author

"Having personally struggled with infertility, I recognize how treatment provides hope, yet is fraught with anxiety and uncertainty, which is why it has become the mission of my practice and life to optimize the experience and maximize the success of all patients yearning to build a family."
— Mark P. Trolice, M.D.

Mark P. Trolice, M.D., FACOG, FACS, FACE, is the director of Fertility CARE: The IVF Center in Orlando, Florida, and Associate Professor in the Department of Obstetrics & Gynecology (OB/GYN) at the University of Central Florida College of Medicine, where he is also the Director of REI for the OB/GYN residency program and for medical students. Dr. Trolice is also the medical director of the egg-banking program at Cryos International.

As a nationally recognized leading fertility specialist, Dr. Trolice has received numerous awards, including the Social Responsibility Award from the National Polycystic Ovary Syndrome Association.

Dr. Trolice is double board-certified in REI and OB/GYN. He maintains annual recertification in these specialties and has been awarded the prestigious American Medical Association's Physicians' Recognition Award annually for many years.

Dr. Trolice is past president of the Florida Society of REI and past division director of REI at Winnie Palmer Hospital for Women & Babies, a division of Orlando Health. His fellow physicians have selected him for Top Doctor in America annually, honoring him as one among the top 5 percent of doctors in the United States, and have named him REI of the Month in the national organization, Fertility Authority.

In 2005, Dr. Trolice was inducted into the prestigious American College of Endocrinology, adding to his unique distinction of also being a fellow in the American College of OB/GYN and the American College of Surgeons.

As part of his commitment to family building, he and his wife, Andrea, fulfilled a lifelong dream when they opened and operated their Angels Among Us adoption agency from 2009 to 2014. For ten years, he directed Fertile Dreams, which he founded as a not-for-profit organization dedicated to increasing fertility awareness and granting scholarships for those unable to afford fertility treatment by sponsoring an annual Paths 2 Parenthood Patient Conference.

Dr. Trolice serves on committees for the American Society for Reproductive Medicine, the Society for Assisted Reproductive Technology, and the Society for Reproductive Endocrinology & Infertility. Dr. Trolice's report of one of his patients—who, at the time, was the oldest woman to give birth using her own egg through IVF—was published in *Fertility and Sterility*.

He serves on the editorial boards of *Ob. Gyn. News* and has served on *The Female Patient*, and *OBG Management*. He appears regularly on television news/talk shows, radio, webcasts, and provides interviews for national newspapers and magazines for breaking reproductive health topics.

Dr. Trolice has authored multiple research studies with publication in leading medical journals and textbooks. He lectures at numerous physician conferences and patient seminars around the country.

His Podcast, "Fertility Health," is nationally recognized and features discussions with reproductive experts on pertinent infertility topics.

Outside of the office, Dr. Trolice has performed with orchestras throughout the country as a jazz vocalist and is an avid marathon runner.

For additional reading, Dr. Trolice can be found on Facebook, Instagram, Twitter, YouTube, LinkedIn, and on the theIVFcenter.com educational blog.

For media inquiries or to schedule Dr. Trolice to speak at your event, please go to MarkTroliceMD.com.

"Every fertility patient has a story to tell. Mine is meant to empower you with knowledge and offer guidance so that one day, hopefully, you may share your story with your child."
— Mark P. Trolice, M.D.

Index

E

eating disorders, 20, 29

ectopic pregnancies, 19, 90, 133, 159–160

EFI (Endometriosis Fertility Index), 104

EGA (estimated gestational age), 42–43, 98, 163

eggs
  age and, 21–22, 40, 42, 63, 69, 195–196
  BCPs (birth control pills) and, 37
  donor eggs, 88, 140, 157, 167, 173, 177, 179, 180
  DOR (diminished ovarian reserve), 21–22, 40, 69
  fertility medications and, 192
  Follicular Phase and, 37
  freezing, 22, 26, 140, 170, 174
  gonadotropins and, 111
  ICSI (intracytoplasmic sperm injection), 62
  IUI (intrauterine insemination) and, 136–137
  IVF (in vitro fertilization) and, 137–138, 197
  Luteal Phase, 38
  multiple pregnancies and, 164
  number of, 40, 69
  ovarian age testing and, 89
  Ovulatory Phase, 37, 126

PGT (preimplantation genetic testing), 35
  retrieval, 137–138, 175, 197
  quality of, 40, 41, 69, 195–196
  sharing, 180
  surrogacy, 141
  tobacco and, 23, 33
  transgender patients, 181, 182
  translocations, 91
  triggering, 130–131

elagolix, 102

electromagnetic radiation, 46, 119

embryos
  chromosomal abnormalities, 91, 97
  chromosomal analysis, 21, 92, 97, 99
  embryo transfer, 138
  endometrial biopsies and, 83
  folic acid and, 97
  freezing, 26, 144, 197
  gonadotropins and, 111
  IVF (in vitro fertilization) transfer, 138, 167
  mosaic embryos, 146
  Müllerian system, 93
  multiple pregnancies, 164, 166
  PGT (preimplantation genetic testing), 26, 35, 92, 99, 143–146, 147
  selecting for IVF (in vitro fertilization), 142
  translocation and, 91

EMD Serono, 153

Endocrine Society, 161

endometrial cancer, 83–84, 94, 99, 108, 126

endometrial dating, 84

endometriomas, 74, 101, 103

endometriosis
  BCPs (birth-control pills) and, 102
  danocrine and, 102
  definition of, 74
  diagnosing, 74, 103
  EFI (Endometriosis Fertility Index), 104
  elagolix, 102
  endometrioma, 103
  GnRH agonist and, 102
  infertility and, 100
  IVF (in vitro fertilization) and, 104
  laparoscopy, 80
  luprolide, 102
  male hormone drugs and, 102
  NNT (number needed to treat), 74
  progestins and, 102
  retrograde menstruation theory, 100–101
  risk factors for, 101
  stages of, 103
  surgical options for, 102, 103
  symptoms of, 67, 101
  treatment options, 74, 102

G

gay male couples, 177, 180

GCs (gestational carriers), 141, 180, 183

gender selection, 137, 145

genetics
  CRISPR (clustered regularly interspaced short palindromic repeats), 148
  family health history, 35
  male infertility and, 114–115
  PGS (preimplantation genetic screening), 144
  PGT (preimplantation genetic testing), 26, 35
  PGT-A (preimplantation genetic testing for aneuploidy), 92, 99, 143–146
  PGT-M (preimplantation genetic testing for monogenic disorders), 147
  RPL (recurrent pregnancy loss) and, 91–92

gestational diabetes, 165

gestational surrogacy, 141

GnRH (gonadotropin-releasing hormone), 105–106

GnRH agonist (gonadotropin-releasing hormone agonist), 102, 130–131, 173

GnRH antagonist (gonadotropin-releasing hormone antagonist), 130, 174

gonadotropins, 76, 102, 110–111, 112, 129, 192

gonorrhea, 18

grants, 151

H

hCG (human chorionic gonadotropin), 38, 130, 159–160

health insurance, 39, 65, 111, 150, 151, 152, 153, 156, 170, 183

hemolytic disease. See Rhesus disease.

heparin, 95, 97

heterotopic pregnancy, 160

holidays, 52

hormones. See individual hormones.

HSG (hysterosalpingogram), 65, 73, 86–87, 87–88, 93, 194

human menopausal gonadotropin, 129

hydrosalpinx, 18, 73, 86

hyperthyroidism, 161

hypothyroidism, 161

hysteroscopy, 93

I

ICI (intracervical insemination), 178

ICSI (intracytoplasmic sperm injection), 62

immunologic testing, 82

individual coping strategies, 53

infertility, definition of, 49, 121, 191. See also secondary infertility.

inositol, 112

insurance, 39, 65, 111, 150, 151, 152, 153, 156, 170, 183

intercourse
  avoiding until ovulation, 24
  optimizing for fertility, 127

International Committee for Monitoring Assisted Reproductive Technologies, 49, 121

intramural fibroids, 75

IP (intended parent), 141

IR (insulin resistance), 108

iron, 31

IUI (intrauterine insemination), 99, 136–137, 178–180, 194–195

IUP (intrauterine pregnancy), 98, 159

IVF (in vitro fertilization)
  AMH (Anti-Müllerian hormone) and, 22
  cancer and, 170
  costs of, 39, 170
  CRISPR (clustered regularly interspaced short palindromic repeats), 148
  embryo selection, 142
  embryo transfer, 138, 167

emergency IVF cycles, 170, 174

endometriosis and, 104

fertility preservation with, 174

Financial Share Program, 158

GCs (gestational carriers) and, 180

gestational surrogacy, 141

guidelines, 167

ICSI (intracytoplasmic sperm injection), 62

insurance and, 170

IUI (intrauterine insemination) and, 99

lesbian couples and, 180

medications, 197

Mediterranean Diet and, 30

metabolomics, 147

non-IVF outcomes compared to, 164

optimizing, 139

overview of, 137–139, 197

PCOS (polycystic ovary syndrome) and, 112

PGT-A (preimplantation genetic testing for aneuploidy) and, 92, 143–146

PGT-M (preimplantation genetic testing for monogenic disorders), 147

repeated cycle of, 63

stress and, 63

success rate of, 26

surrogacy and, 177

TESA (testicular sperm aspiration), 62

time-lapse photography, 147

twin pregnancies, 177

IVF Financial Share Program, 158

L

laparoscopic surgery, 79, 80, 193–194

lesbian couples, 178–180

letrozole, 61, 110, 112, 129, 192

LGBTQ patients

adoption, 182

equality, 183

gay male couples, 180

insurance and, 183

lesbian couples, 178–179

transgender couples, 182

transgender men, 181

LH (luteinizing hormone), 24, 37, 38, 89, 106, 118, 129, 131

LightStream, 156

loans against assets, 151

LOD (laparoscopic ovarian diathermy), 61, 76, 110, 111, 112

lubricants, 127

luprolide, 102

Luteal Phase, 38, 84, 96

M

male infertility

age and, 22, 48, 71, 88

azoospermia, 45, 72, 115, 116–118

CBAVD (congenital bilateral absence of the vas deferens), 114

cryptorchidism, 118

elevated FSH/LH, 118

evaluation, 196

FSH (follicle stimulating hormone), 118

genetics and, 114–115

health and, 45

LH (luteinizing hormone), 118

lifestyle and, 45, 120

NOA (non-obstructive azoospermia), 117

OA (obstructive azoospermia), 117

obesity and, 72

RE (retrograde ejaculation), 116–117

statistics, 40, 113

TESA (testicular sperm aspiration), 62, 117

testosterone and, 72, 119

varicocele, 116

vasectomy reversal, 118

YCMD (Y chromosome microdeletion), 115

O

OA (obstructive azoospermia), 117

OBD (oil-based dye), 87

obesity, 20, 29–30, 45, 72, 108

OHSS (ovarian hyperstimulation syndrome), 111, 133–134

OMDs (Oriental Medical Doctors), 123

oncofertility, 169

OPK (ovulation predictor kit), 14, 24, 37, 67, 126, 136, 179

OSA (obstructive sleep apnea), 107

ovaries
    cancer treatment and, 132, 170–171, 172
    chemotherapy and, 170, 172
    DOR (diminished ovarian reserve), 40
    estradiol and, 36
    menstrual irregularities and, 29
    ovarian age tests, 39–43, 69, 88–89
    ovarian diathermy 61, 76
    ovarian drilling, 107
    ovarian stimulation, 130, 136, 164, 174
    ovarian torsion, 134
    radiation shielding, 175
    tissue freezing, 175

over-the-counter remedies, 123

ovulation
    blockers, 130
    Cycle Day One, 36
    DOR (diminished ovarian reserve), 40
    eggs and, 40, 179
    evaluation and, 67
    Female Athlete Triad and, 20
    Follicular Phase, 37, 69
    hormones and, 105–106
    induction, 61, 110–112, 128–129, 164, 192
    intercourse timing and, 24, 127
    IUI (intrauterine insemination) and, 136
    letrozole and, 61
    LOD (laparoscopic ovarian diathermy), 111
    Luteal Phase, 38, 84, 96
    OPK (ovulation predictor kit), 14, 24, 37, 67, 126, 136, 179
    optimizing for fertility, 126–127
    ovarian diathermy, 61
    overview of, 36
    Ovulatory Phase, 37, 126
    PCOS (polycystic ovary syndrome) and, 61, 75–76, 106, 110–111
    predicting, 67
    progesterone and, 65, 83, 84
    specialist training and, 79
    timing of, 38
    weight and, 20

P

PCOS (polycystic ovary syndrome)
    anxiety and, 112
    BCPs (birth-control pills) and, 61, 112
    depression and, 112
    diagnosing, 76, 106
    endometrial biopsy and, 83
    endometrial cancer and, 108
    gonadotropins and, 110–111, 112
    hormone imbalance and, 106
    inositol and, 112
    IVF (in vitro fertilization) and, 112
    letrozole and, 112, 192
    LOD (laparoscopic ovarian diathermy) and, 112
    management of, 109
    medical risks of, 109
    menstrual cycle and, 67
    Metabolic Syndrome, 108, 109
    metformin and, 112
    miscarriage and, 107
    OPK (ovulation predictor kit) and, 37
    OSA (obstructive sleep apnea) and, 107
    overview of, 75–76
    ovulation and, 61, 75–76, 106, 110–111

U

unilateral orchiectomy, 71

UPT (urine pregnancy test), 38, 130

uterine septum, 93

uterine transplantation, 175–176

V

vaccinations, 34

vaginal bleeding, 162–163

vaginal lubricants, 127

validation, 57

varicocele, 46, 116, 139

vasectomy, 58, 62, 118

vitamins, 31, 32

W

WCD (water contrast dye), 87

weight
  BMI (body mass index), 20, 68, 99, 108, 109, 110, 123
  Female Athlete Triad, 20, 29, 67, 188–189
  obesity, 20, 29–30, 45, 72, 108
  PCOS (polycystic ovary syndrome) and, 107, 112

WHO (World Health Organization), 49, 114, 183, 191

WINFertility, 154

WINFertilityRx, 154

women's health
  calcium, 31
  diet, 29–30
  family health history, 35
  iron, 31
  medical conditions, 33
  Mediterranean Diet, 30
  minerals, 31
  preconception check-ups, 29
  vitamins, 31, 32

Y

YCMD (Y chromosome microdeletion), 115